Sweet
Invisible
Body

sweet invisible body

reflections

on a life

with

diabetes

Lisa Roney

Henry Holt and Company

New York

Henry Holt and Company, LLC
Publishers since 1866
115 West 18th Street
New York, New York 10011

Henry Holt® is a registered trademark of
Henry Holt and Company, LLC.

Published in Canada by Fitzhenry & Whiteside Ltd.,
195 Allstate Parkway, Markham, Ontario L3R 4T8.

Grateful acknowledgment is made to the following for
permission to reprint previously published material:

Terrestrials by Paul West. Reprinted with the permission of Scribner, a Division of
Simon and Schuster, from *Terrestrials* by Paul West. Copyright © 1997 by Paul West.

A Death in the Family by James Agee. Copyright © 1957 by The James Agee Trust,
renewed 1985 by Mia Agee. Used by permission of Grosset & Dunlap, Inc.,
a division of Penguin Putnam Inc.

Giants in the Earth by O. E. Rölvaag. Copyright © 1927 by Harper & Row
Publishers, Inc. Renewed 1955 by Jennie Marie Berdahl Rölvaag.
Reprinted by permission of HarperCollins Publishers, Inc.

Library of Congress Cataloging-in-Publication Data
Roney, Lisa.
Sweet invisible body : reflections on a life with
diabetes / Lisa Roney.
p.   cm.
ISBN 0-8050-5625-4 (hc. : alk. paper)
1. Roney, Lisa—Health.   2. Diabetics—United States—
Biography.   I. Title.
RC660.4.R66   1999   98-51819
362.1'96462'0092—dc21   CIP
[b]

Henry Holt books are available for special promotions
and premiums. For details contact: Director, Special Markets.

First Edition 1999

Designed by Michelle McMillian

Printed in the United States of America
All first editions are printed on acid-free paper. ∞

1 3 5 7 9 10 8 6 4 2

To Paul, with deep gratitude,
and in memory of Cassie Marie and Stella Rondo,
who, though wordless, were with me every day

contents

Acknowledgments

Paul West must always come first and last in any list of those I thank for support in my endeavors as a writer. Without him, I might never have found my voice; with him, I have been challenged, befriended, prodded, proffered, and very well taught. My debt to him would fill the sky.

To my other writing teachers I also express my gratitude for their insights and support, especially to Peter Schneeman, who has remained a friend and consultant long after our official professional relationship ended. Many of my graduate school peers have also taught me a great deal and have listened to endless confused versions of the stories that appear in this book. Deep, deep gratitude and love go to Sally Pont, who read the first garbled draft of the first chapter and set me on course with her comments and empathy. To the other members of my former writers' group—Ann, Mary, Joann, Gigi, Lisa, Lorena, and Marguerite—I also extend my thanks for the ways they helped me become a better writer, though we had dissolved before this project came to fruition. Thanks also to Suzanne Marcum for reading some chapters and to Mara Gorman for expressing faith in my abilities.

My many other friends and associates I thank for their indulgence and understanding during the past months of my self-absorption in this project. I am grateful to those colleagues who have been supportive of my dual career, especially to my current advisor, Susan Squier, Brill Professor of English and Women's Studies at Penn State University, and the members of my dissertation group—Holly, Christina, Julie, and Harvey. I'm sorry that I can't name all of the friends who have been encouraging, but I am especially indebted to Susan Reider, Anita Katter, Craig Irvine, John Spooner, Mark Hersh, Carolyn Bershad, and all those who participated in selecting the title.

In addition, I would like to thank my family of writers—my great-grandfather, Thomas Jefferson Campbell, whom I never met, but whose two slim books set a standard in our house; my Grandmother Meek, who penned sweet poems; my mother, Anne Meek, who penned fiercer poems and guided me in all my early writing with an unerring sense of grammar and vocabulary; my brother, Kelly, for his unstinting admiration and discussion of details; and my father, Robert Roney, not only for his pride in my writing but also for always buying me new running shoes.

Many thanks to my physician, Jan Ulbrecht, both for helping to keep me healthy for the past twelve years and for reading the entire manuscript with a careful eye toward accuracy, as well as with his characteristic willingness to learn and understand.

My editor, Tracy Brown, and all the other kindly souls at Henry Holt have been a pleasure to work with, and I thank them for their respect and competence. Likewise, I'd like to thank my ·

agent, Elaine Markson, and her former assistant, Pari Berk, as well as Charis Conn at *Harper's*, for their willingness to invest in me and their belief in the quality and content of my work. And that brings me back around to Paul, who introduced me to them, in addition to the joy of letting loose in language.

May we all thrive together.

Prologue:
Looking for Lost Time

If you do not tell the truth about yourself you cannot
tell it about other people.
　　　　　　—Virginia Woolf, "The Leaning Tower"

The first thing I remember from one day this past summer is
standing at my dresser, where I keep my glucose meter, and seeing
Leslee nearby, peering tentatively through the door. I knew that
her presence embarrassed me, but I could not figure out what
Leslee was doing there. In fact, it surprised me to be standing up,
as the last thing in my mind was curling under the covers of my
bed, and the sensation of awakening in this vertical position rendered me dizzy, unsettled. As in a dream, I wondered if I might be
naked and looked down on my silly pink pajamas with relief.
Then I glanced at the jumble of items on my dresser, but they,
too, made no sense to me. Wasn't I supposed to know how to
operate this little machine? But I didn't, and my hands fluttered
uselessly in front of me.

Leslee beckoned me to come downstairs to the kitchen and
get some juice, which I obediently did in my state of blurred

numbness, following along like a sleepy child and collapsing into a chair at the kitchen table while Leslee poured and handed me a large glass of shining golden liquid. Intermittently, my head would droop to my arm on the tabletop, as though magnetized, the weight of gravity pulling at me as though there were no other force in the universe, but Leslee would remind me, "Drink some more," and soon enough I was coming back around. Norepine-phrine, an adrenaline-like hormone released when the blood sugar falls too low, pulsed through my system, and along with comprehending what had happened, I began shaking and freez-ing and chattering. There was, in a remote region of my mind, an awareness that I should shut up, but I launched into a long discourse on the cacti in the greenhouse window. Leslee and I often talked about such domestic topics as houseplants, but this almost normal conversation was lopsided and eerie under the circumstances. On and on I rambled, with Leslee occasion-ally interrupting to ask if I felt better now. Gradually, I grew qui-eter, and we sat at the kitchen table in silence, my hands trembling slightly, Leslee adrift in a patient uncertainty about my condition.

The phone jangled its interruption—my mother calling to see if order had been restored. "Yes, yes," I told her. "Leslee got me up. It's fine, fine."

"I called twice before," she said, relating her own traumatic experience. "The first time you answered the phone, but weren't making any sense." I could hear the anxiety twisting her voice. "The second time you didn't answer at all."

"I'm sorry," I said.

Leslee reported that when she'd first arrived, thrown into action by a subsequent call by my mother, she thought she'd found me not so bad off. Not wanting to intrude on the privacy of my bedroom, she'd called to me from the doorway, telling me to get up. To her satisfaction, I did, and went straight to the dresser and the glucose meter.

In the next moments, however, she realized that there was no plastic strip in the machine and that I had not pricked my finger after all. She had seen me perform this test enough times out at lunch that she knew I wasn't doing it properly. The meter's series of beeps permeated the air emptily, and my hands hung loose by my sides. My eyes were blank.

"You were going through the motions," she said, shaking her head in wonder, "but you were definitely not there."

Although Leslee and I had known each other for some time, she was unprepared for what she might encounter. Although she, like several other friends, had agreed to be on call in such cases, I had never really explained in full detail what I might be like when severely hypoglycemic, and Leslee had never seen me this way before. Most of the time I wake myself, scramble out of bed to the refrigerator, and manage before I conk out again to down enough juice to ensure my recovery. During times when I'm out in public, I keep close tabs on my glucose levels and whenever they dip I take care of it as quickly and unobtrusively as possible. I keep my lows to myself, so even my good friends rarely see any effects from them, and, besides, the variability of the condition eludes explanation. Sometimes I get the shakes pretty early in the process or feel my heart pounding strangely—things no one else need notice—and pop a few glucose tablets in my mouth, recover almost immediately, and never miss a beat. Other times, I get no sign until my vision clouds with pulsing speckles or I find myself suddenly unable to read or to speak the word that lurks like a wildcat on the edge of my consciousness. Even then, other people can't see what is happening—I usually look all right, though eventually I ramble, say weird and often funny things, and grow uncoordinated. My body often flips into automatic pilot, good in that I often help myself by getting juice or food without really knowing what I'm doing, but bad in that I hide my condition from others who might help me earlier, keep me from getting behind the wheel of a car, prevent me from wasting twenty or more minutes of a class I'm trying and failing to teach, or simply understand why I'm acting oddly.

Luckily, I am not usually violent, as some people are, though there have been times when I've flailed and punched—once at my mother, once at an old college friend who had to whisk me to the emergency room, more than once at lovers in the wee morning hours. A team of cops nearly strangled my friend Mike once, when he'd run wildly hypoglycemic through the streets proclaiming that he was pursued by murderous political fanatics and pulling along a stranger in his wake, trying to save her. Despite the fact that by the time the police arrived, Mike's wife Daphne had caught up to him and explained his condition, they remained certain he was on drugs and deserved to be punished as well as subdued. Another diabetic acquaintance of mine once grew so crazed that when he regained consciousness in the hospital he'd had a shoulder broken in the melee. Such stories abound among diabetics, part of an amazement we have about losing ourselves so completely from time to time. We love to tell them because they are often funny and almost always bizarre, and because we can regain the moments by talking about them as though we were there, as though we had been watching along with our friends and family. However, I sometimes pause at the depth of low blood sugar's unpleasantness from my own internal perspective. There is just about no condition I can think of that I hate more. Is this, I wonder, what it's like to be psychotic, to have multiple personalities, to move in and out of reality? How does it compare to having a tumor gradually shutting down various parts of the brain? Why does my heart feel as though it will burst, stop, leap into my toes, flutter like a bird hit by a car? Will there be a time when I punch someone hard trying to clear the hallucinatory midges from my field of vision?

Fortunately, I hadn't tried to smack Leslee. Still, she was shaken, perhaps even more than I. After all, even though most of my friends and family have seen few of these episodes, and some have never witnessed even one, I have been through many.

"It's always weird to see, the first time," I said to her. "I'm sorry."

And so, even though I adore sleeping, long for it like a fleeting lover, I usually do so only tentatively, skimming on the surface out of fear of not waking again, stirring from dreams that never resolve themselves, like some new mother listening for her baby's fragile breath. I try to remain aware of myself while I sleep because it is then, during the stillness of eight—or seven—or six hours' slumber, that my body is most vulnerable to these hideous lows. Though my doctor reassures me that, aside from situations related to alcohol and automobiles, few people actually die of hypoglycemia because the insulin eventually subsides on its own, these episodes shame and haunt me, the most apparent shadow on my semblance of a normal life.

Diabetes affects almost everything a person does—the insulin injections are the least of it, though they are tiresome. If I could take my three shots a day, if the same daily dosage worked just fine—like with heart, blood pressure, thyroid pills—then I'd be happy as a clam. Diabetes, however, is a constant balancing act, with adjustments of insulin dosage, constant calculations about food and exercise, about whether a given interaction is worth the energy, about the timing of every walk, jog, movie, lecture, air-line flight, nap, phone conversation, and meal.

Yet diabetes is invisible. No one can tell that I have it just by looking at me. No one experiences it as serious or catastrophic because it doesn't have the dramatic nature of cancer, heart attack, or more apparent disabilities. For fifteen or twenty years, even I did not think of it as debilitating, so I certainly don't con-demn others for not realizing. Rather, I have developed the habit of explaining, telling endless stories about my disease, asking for a modicum of sympathy that I insist never grow maudlin or pity-ing, for I couldn't bear that. It is definitely worse to be treated as a martyr than for my problem to be ignored, and the fine tight-rope is hard for people to walk.

Once I attended a potluck dinner party that turned into a chaotic bash attended by more than fifty people with mounds of food and piles of coats competing for space in several rooms of a local boardinghouse. Discreetly, I slipped into a back room to take my insulin, but another woman had followed me in, looking for the cigarettes in her coat pocket. She freaked at the sight of my needle.

"Oh, my God," she said, "why are you doing that in here? I can't look. I could never do that." Her entire body recoiled in fear and repulsion.

"Yes, you could," I began in explanation.

"No!" She would hear none of it. "I hate shots." She moved quickly away toward the door.

"You'd be dead, then," I said in parting, hating her naïveté.

Certainly, I'd rather my friends think nothing of it than flee in such silly fright, and much of my life I've spent reassuring them that it is no big deal in order not to scare them off forever. This, however, means that I've denied my own fears and exhaustion, my own hatred of the necessary routine and despair at the uncertainty of my future health. On the one hand, that has provided me with a wonderfully normal life. After my diagnosis, I went back to school immediately with no special dispensation; I continued riding horses through woods and fields; I swam in the neighbor's pool; I spent nights at friends' homes and weeks at the homes of my friends on the other side of the state. Later, I went far away to college, went backpacking in the wilderness, traveled the country, strolled through blizzards, drank plenty of beer, and kept volume after volume of a journal in which my diabetes is hardly mentioned. No one, least of all me, thought of me as ill. The fact is, however, that I am both ill and healthy, supposed opposites that we often have trouble holding in our minds at once. I need to be able to hold both these self-images together, or I cannot know myself.

None of us can determine how our lives *might* have gone if this or that had never happened, and likewise I cannot know what my life would be like had I never become a diabetic. It happened one traumatic year—which I think of as The Year—in which I also (before the diabetes) broke two bones in a fall from my horse and spent six weeks in a wheelchair and (after the diabetes) began menstruating and lost my beloved grandfather to a brain tumor. My family had just moved cross-state, leaving my friends and secure social roles behind, and I was lonely and miserable both before and after the physical calamities began to fall. I was eleven, then twelve years old, with nothing to do with my anguish and confusion. I've been working it out ever since.

This book is the result of trying, over the past few years, to come to a balance between optimism and pessimism, between what is normal and average in me and what is different and difficult. We all face such contradictions in our lives and personalities. We all must confront the "what if"s, the missed opportunities, the boulders that have fallen on our tender limbs, twisting and breaking some permanently, determining over time the shape our growth takes. My own long-buried feelings about being given a life sentence at the age of eleven have emerged gradually, in the same kind of process of self-discovery that we all go through as we grow up, mature, and face the parameters of our lives. We all want to know who we are and why we are who we are, and diabetes has provided for me both self and cause. I try to sort out the diabetes from the rest of me, but it is impossible. It does not erase the other aspects of my experience and personality, but infuses them all with its bittersweet taste. Each of us has such identity markers, and what they are is not so important as how we explore them, how we acknowledge both their effect and the ways in which we as individuals reach beyond them.

For we do reach beyond them. That, too, is what these stories are about: trying to show in detail what it is that I have found in my experience and in my head, trying to emphasize that our differences are fascinating rather than merely alienating, that if we look the strangeness in the eye, it may become familiar.

A word about memory: I have written nothing in this book that I don't remember. I have not made up anecdotes or descriptions. I quote people saying the precise words I remember their saying, but I do not have these conversations on tape. As we all know by now, memory is not absolute, and I make no claims that this book represents any objective truth. Others will certainly remember some things differently. Others who have diabetes will have had experiences very unlike mine. It is my hope that these variations in memory and experience may become not nasty quibbles, but part of the world's dialogue about the meanings of illness, health, family, friendship, love, and language. For we must be forever starting over with talking, telling our truths, and listening to each other in order to make sense of our lives. No one else can do it for us.

Sweet
Invisible
Body

part one

Farewell

to Chess Pie

and Other

Tennessee

Habits

We are talking now of summer evenings in Knoxville, Tennessee, in the time that I lived there so
successfully disguised to myself as a child.
                    —James Agee, A Death in the Family

The French blue kitchen of my grandparents' house on Moody Avenue in Martin, Tennessee, is only part of a pile of scavenged rubble now, but it was one of my favorite places as a child. On special occasions, we ate in the dining room, but most of the time food appeared on the cracked pink willow plates on the Formica table in the alcove lined with windows at the back of the kitchen. My grandmother's tremulous voice would call us in from a game of croquet under the trees in the backyard, and we would cram around the table, jostling elbow to elbow to get to the fried chicken, the cornbread, the creamed fresh corn from my grandfather's garden, and the conversation.

"Did I ever tell you how my brother Russell lost the ends of the fingers of his right hand?" my grandfather might ask, winking at my brother and me because we knew my grandmother would protest this sort of gruesome story.

"Now, Paul," she would say, but the pleasure would flood her face, just as it did when my grandfather let go of the steering wheel to clap his hands together as we drove down the highway. Though we did not shriek with excitement here, as we did in the car, my brother and I were aware that our grandparents performed this ritual of titillation and admonition for us. Both were playing roles they relished, and the contradictions were designed to teach us something.

"Tell us, tell us," my brother and I would chime, and my mother would egg him on with a question about just how long ago it was that this tragedy had befallen Russell. "I never remember him having those fingertips," she might say.

I had hardly known my great-uncle Russell, but his had been the first funeral I'd attended, and the casket had been open so I remembered him well. I remembered the church, clapboard on a concrete block foundation, smack out in the middle of a field gone brown with summer drought. The heat had been palpable, waves of it billowing from the tin roof as we followed the dust rising behind the line of cars to the ceremony. The lights inside the church were bright, and funeral-home fans—round disks of printed cardboard mounted on wide Popsicle-like sticks—filled the air with waving motion and whispering sound, but not with a breeze. Ladies in hats and gloves perspired through their summer dresses, and men mopped their brows mournfully with yellowed handkerchiefs. As we filed past Uncle Russell's body on the way out, people touched him, spoke to him, and sobbed for breath.

To me, he had looked like a figure in the wax museum, his flannel and overalls replaced with a gray suit, his large ears and long face as unreal as Abe Lincoln's, his beat-up hands stilled at his sides. Were his fingertips missing at the funeral? I had not noticed, and I could not imagine he had ever been young, but here my grandfather was, telling a story that featured Russell as a child. At age five, my grandfather told us, Russell insisted on playing a game of patty-cake on the chopping block where their older sister Effie hammered idly with the hatchet.

"Stop, Ef," little Russell said, putting his hand out to make it happen, "and play with me."

"Quit it," she replied. "I'm busy. Now get your fingers outta the way."

Back and forth they went, Russell sticking out his hand over and over to interrupt Effie's chopping, Effie pausing to yell at him to move his hand and then going ahead with her gouging of the wood. She grew more and more annoyed and finally said, "Now this time I really mean it. Get your hand outta there." Russell paused one turn, and then flung his hand back into the midst of Effie's new rhythm. In one smooth motion, she chopped off the ends of his two middle fingers.

In the blue kitchen, we would laugh and shake our heads at Russell's stubbornness and Effie's meanness. The loss of his fingertips was no longer a tragedy, as he had gone on to a long and full life as a farmer and landowner. Effie, always flamboyant and strong-willed, was long dead. Their personalities, however, still offered us all kinds of lessons. Respect danger. Pay attention to what people tell you. Don't fight over stupid issues. It takes two to tango. And horrible events are to be overcome, set aside, even made fun of.

Mostly farmers, my people had a Protestant work ethic as wide open as the Mississippi Delta and as craggy as the Appalachian Mountains from which they drew their livings. My great-grandfather Campbell had been a newspaperman and my great-grandmother Craddock, after her divorce, had run a beauty salon in her apartment, but they, too, reflected the insistent drive toward work, toward endeavor, toward making good. They were a tough, practical people, and my sense of this grew over the years of my childhood, as my parents, brother, and I drove back and forth across the long state of Tennessee, moving and visiting.

Tennessee is a green and beautiful place, traversed by ugly Interstate 40, from the eastern mountains and valleys, across the fine, high Cumberland Plateau, to the flat, steamy, rich-soiled river bottoms of the western half of the state. The regions are so distinct that when I was a child, the signs at the state borders said, WELCOME TO THE THREE STATES OF TENNESSEE. My family lived divided between east and west, and we spent a lot of time on the highway, driving past tumble-down barns, mud-flecked beasts, rusted-out trucks and tractors, ruined farmhouses, creeping kudzu vines, and cemeteries. One of our favorite car games was cow-counting, but the numbers never went very high, as every one of the frequent cemeteries we passed would reduce one competitor's score to zero.

We were fond of cemeteries, however, and often used them for picnicking when no park was available. My grandfather, in particular, liked to take us around to our relatives' graves and tell us stories about them there, as though the stones with their names and dates could make the stories even more real, more affecting. His favorite, Freeman Cemetery, sat nestled in trees just a mile or so down the road from his sister Charlie's house and adjacent to the farm still run by his cousin Dillard—a century farm, in the family for over a hundred years—and so it was a natural stop in tours of memory lane. We drove by the house he'd been born in, and the church he'd attended—the same one in my precious photograph of my grandfather as a teenager, sitting in a buggy behind his first horse, a dapple gray named Maud—before arriving at the graveyard to pull away weeds, make sure the markers were upright, and listen to tales: how my great-grandfather Felix tried to teach his wife, Temp, to read; how Uncle John came home from the war to die a slow death; how my own grandfather had missed being at Vanderbilt with the Fugitives because of a bad crop. These times, and most of the people in them, were long gone, but stories, we learned from him, allowed you to live forever.

I often have wondered what stories my grandfather might have fashioned out of my illness, but I had been diagnosed with diabetes less than a year when he died of a brain tumor. He and my grandmother came from Martin to Memphis for the surgery, and before going to the hospital, he, still tall and athletic at seventy-four, sat in the rocking chair in the living room trying to tell me something. I could tell it was important and listened patiently as he leaned forward and patted my arm emphatically. But he could not tell me. The tumor had already begun to interfere with his language function, and his sentences came out garbled. There was no story to transform the tragedy into experience, and there was no medical treatment that could repair my grandfather to his former self. He went home in a casket, silenced.

A couple of years later, the newspapers ran a different kind of illness story. The state was suing the parents of a girl my age in order to force medical care for a cancerous tumor in the girl's thigh. Hardscrabble fundamentalists, the family did not put stock in medicine. If the girl's faith were strong enough and the Lord heard their prayers, they said, she would recover. If not, God had some other plan.

For months, the lawyers argued in court, the piles of motions rising like the growth in the girl's leg. A photo showed her with cavernous shadows under her eyes, a weak smile, and a long, dark skirt covering her body. The newspapers reported that the tumor had reached the size of a football before it was removed. By then, the cancer had metastasized. A couple of weeks after the court-ordered surgery, the girl was dead. The debate, however, raged on for some time, her legacy.

Loving the piney smell of my mountains, the fierce thunderstorms that electrified my southern atmosphere, and the long, low sounds of cicadas in the summertime, I nonetheless wondered what this land had wrought. It seemed full of kooks and fanatics. As yet unfamiliar with New England Gothic, Pennsylvania Dutch perversion, Minnesota Chippewa degradation, and West Coast schizophrenia, I thought all the rednecks and crazy people were in the South. All the death, too. I was a little bit embarrassed about where I was from, especially when there was any hint of Holy Roller or Dolly Parton. Still, I wondered about the fundamentalist girl's bravery, pure and past, and compared it sometimes to my messy ongoing struggle.

Nostalgia already infected me, through an innocent girl's martyrdom, through my grandfather's stories, through cemetery genealogies, through the recipes passed down, many of them faded and out of reach by the time I was twelve. At ten I had earned my Girl Scout badge in cooking, and part of the task involved collecting family recipes. Well, anyone could fry a chicken or put together a batch of biscuits, but the sweets in my family—they were stupendous.

Grandmother Meek was famed for both her fine, white coconut cake and her East Tennessee dried apple stack cake. Her divinity candy shone like angel wings and melted on your tongue like a snowflake. Grandmother Roney boasted the original and fragrant amalgamation cake with its rich yellow frosting full of nuts, raisins, and coconut. She could make a buttery fudge that made your teeth hurt, it was so intense. But it had been my step-grandmother, Billie, who had sent me a recipe not only rich, wonderful, and rooted in the South, but also simple enough for a beginner to make: chess pie, a smooth confection that tastes like the sun on the first day of the year it turns the trees golden.

I tapped the sugar into the glass bowl, measured out a little cornmeal, vanilla, and vinegar, watched the butter melting in its enamel pan. Then I cracked the eggs into the mixture, popped the whole thing into the oven, and waited to take it out, a miraculously thickened custard, barely browned around the edges and as light on the tongue as a whisper. Although for the requisite scout badge dinner I had used a store-bought crust, my family beamed.

At ten, chess pie was my triumph. At twelve, a now impossible past. My mother taught me to make whole wheat bread instead.

There was a whole new recipe for life, however, that yielded no edible product, no matter how prosaic. I tapped the tablet into the test tube, measured the urine drop by drop, charted the color of the bubbling liquid in this new recipe of diabetes care. I knocked the air from the syringe, popped it into my leg, withdrew it efficiently. I did what had to be done, no more, no less, in one family tradition I could still maintain: practical perseverance.

They used to tease that I was fourteen going on fifty.

1

Pretty Ugly

My mother didn't want me to let my hair grow, but I insisted. At five years old, living in a new town with no new friends, I wanted to be like Patsy, my favorite baby-sitter back in Memphis. If I could be like Patsy, with her long, shiny brown hair pulled into a neat ponytail, her eyes round and sweet as root beer candies, her legs below her pleated skirt tan and smooth like the surface of my mother's creamy coffee, then maybe I would have some friends here in Knoxville.

And, so, over my mother's protests, I began to let my own blond locks descend. I think my mother thought I would give it up, that it would be another child's whim gone tomorrow. Indeed, when the hair began to flip and curl in strange ways around my chin, I was annoyed. But in a little girl, it doesn't take much to reach the ponytail stage. I had to learn to braid it myself, by feel behind my head, because my mother said that if I wanted the hair, then I had to take care of it. I practiced on the fringes of the white chenille bedspread at my grandparents', and soon enough, though my hair would never stay in firm, tight ropes, I got the hang of it. My growing collection of barrettes— two turquoise Scottie dogs, a brass clasp enameled with three red roses, an old silver oval of my grandmother's, several plastic clips from the dime store—and assorted ribbons and elasticized bands filled a plastic box that had come containing shower curtain hooks. They were my first cosmetic concern, and I soon developed a love-hate relationship with them.

In fact, I liked them all as objects and I loved fingering the box's contents, lining them up on the dresser, and matching them to my socks. But I hated wearing them in my hair. The elastic bands and barrettes simply wouldn't stay. My hair, fine and wispy, escaped around the edges, and the ornaments fell out. My braids looked like shaggy caterpillars, my bangs would fall straight over my forehead with a barrette flapping between my eyes, and the ribbons would slide toward the back of my head. The ribbons were the worst, and my mother and I battled over them for years. I always preferred to wear my hair loose, but she wanted me to keep my hair out of my face and before school every morning would tie a narrow ribbon, bow on top, behind my ears. They pinched, they looked stupid, and I always took them out and slipped them into my book bag on the way to school. Sometimes I would forget to put them back on before I went home, and my mother would sigh and shake her head.

When you are a child, beauty is such a simple thing—no makeup, anti-wrinkle cream, hair dye, hair removal, or surgery required. In spite of my mother's worry about the hair hanging in my face, I had confidence in the beauty of my hair all by itself. I was the darling of both my grandfathers, who praised my cuteness on every visit. My second-grade schoolteacher, in a thank-you note for a scarf I'd given her at the end of the year, wrote, "Each time I wear it, I'll think of a pretty, little girl who does such fine work in school. . . ." Compared to my cousin Rebecca, who was always rubbing her puffy eyes and allergy-red nose into tormented shapes, I was angelic without even trying.

I would get my comeuppance. But even before that would happen, I had begun struggling with beauty. I wanted long hair, but I also wanted to wear pointed-toe shoes, not the practical saddle-oxfords my mother forced on me. A few years later when saddle-oxfords became all the rage in my middle school, I had my first realization of the arbitrary nature of beauty standards, an inkling that no one could ever get purchase in the shifting sands of fashion and in the quicksand of unrealistic cultural ideals. I lived, after all, not only in the larger consumption-driven culture of the United States, but more specifically in a South where many women and girls still wouldn't leave the house "without my face on." During high school summers, my friend Susan would apply her makeup before our 7 A.M. jogs, because we might stop by the grocery store for a bottle of juice afterward. At seventeen, she couldn't afford to be seen sans mascara, eyeliner, foundation, and lipstick. She didn't feel herself without them.

My childhood was characterized by my mother's ambivalence about all of this. Many years later, after my parents' divorce when I was twenty-four, my mother would renounce the feminism of personal habits to become a high-heeled, sculpted-nails clotheshorse, but when I was small she was an attractive but low-key professional educator, dressed for the public school trenches without any makeup. Looking back, I realize that she never cultivated any of that sort of femininity in me, never taught me how to apply eye shadow, never curled my hair, never gave me jewelry.

I think my mother, only twenty when she first became pregnant and with two children by age twenty-three, wasn't even used to her own adult body, and, of course, she wanted to avoid the mistakes her own parents had made. Her own mother had made her aware from a young age of how her own body was a commodity for marriage. Scratched across the cheek during a neighborhood scramble at age eight or nine, my mother was admonished that she must rub the wound with Vaseline twice a day in order to avoid a permanent scar. Such a disfigured face, her mother said, might prevent anyone from falling in love with and marrying her.

Not wanting to inflict such strictures and fears on me, my mother let my body grow like honeysuckle over a back lot fence—strong and unfettered, but also undisciplined, untended, and basically ignored. I ran hard with my brother and our friends, first in the sandbox and backyard, later exploring the nearby woods and playing "night games" of Kick the Can and Capture the Flag. But my parents only reluctantly taught us how to swim and how to ride bikes. My mother insisted I have short-term tap-dancing lessons, but we never danced at home. Though we enjoyed a good meal, a hike in the mountains, the purring presence of a cat, we were a rather cerebral family.

As with swimming and bike riding, I always felt behind when it came to style and grooming. When I went to my mother to ask about shaving my legs, after having the difference pointed out to me at the local swimming pool, she told me I was too young. It was my step-grandmother who gave me my first razor for Christmas one year. There was no ear-piercing, no bottle of lavender nail polish, no poster of Donny Osmond on the wall. I didn't start wearing bras until a boy at school had run his finger down my back and commented that my boobs were swinging free. I went home and tearfully reported the incident to my mother, and, with her apologies, we went immediately to the department store.

It was the fall of 1971, just before my broken bones and my diabetes. My family was back in Memphis, and I had left behind my rough-and-tumble friends in Knoxville for the ultimately conservative social atmosphere of the real South, untempered by the presence of East Tennessee mountains. Tomboys were not tolerated, and the girls in my school already had a growing interest in the opinions of boys.

The "foundations" department at Goldsmith's spread across half of the entire second floor, and my mother and I rode the escalator right into a land of lace, satin, and spandex. A plump, gray-haired lady packed into her dark blue suit minced her way over to us, moving tightly between the overladen racks and within the obviously great compression of her own underwear. I cringed at her discomfort. She smiled hungrily.

"We're here for her first bra," my mother whispered conspiratorially.

The woman appraised me kindly. "Well, we can fix you right up, sugar," she said. "It's so exciting—you'll be prettier than ever."

Embarrassed, I milled through the lacy, heavily padded, variously colored bras hanging on racks, while my mother and the saleslady selected several "training" bras in cardboard boxes. I tugged at the elastic bands of my sleeves and scratched idly at the red welts they always left on my arms. What would it be like wearing elastic around my chest all the time? Did the tiny swelling of my breasts really merit this?

In the dressing room, I tried on several of the thin, unthreatening training bras. They weren't bad, and, surprisingly, I liked the sense of protection they gave me. My mother showed me how to lean forward, to let my small breasts fall into and fill the cups, and handed me each bra as she took it out of its box. We didn't talk much, but in the next cubicle, a drama took place.

"It hurts, Mama," a girl's voice whined. "I don't want to wear it."

She sounded about my age, perhaps a little older, and I thought at first she was talking about a bra. Some of the ones out there had looked pretty tough—rigorously shaped, with hard wires around the bottom of each cup, with straps so thin they looked cutting, and bands so wide that it took three or four hooks to keep them secured. But then her mother spoke.

"I won't have you jiggling all over the place. No proper young lady can do without a girdle, and you might as well get used to it now."

"But, Mama . . ."

"No buts about it. If you want to get a larger size, then fine. We can face up to how fat you are. But you're going to wear a girdle. I want no more arguments."

"Very old-fashioned," my mother said on our way out of the dressing room, probably in answer to the horrified look on my face. "Don't worry. You'll never have to wear one of those." In spite of the fact that I'd wanted a bra, we were together on the matter of girdles. No matter how plump you got, too much bodily discipline of that sort seemed horrible, somehow sick.

I might get annoyed that my mother ignored my developing body, but at least that allowed me to roll happily in the leaves with my dog, to run wide circles through the long grass, to rise over the double oxer on the back of my horse, to never question that connection between the idea and the execution of a physical act. With my fall from the horse in December 1971, my physical confidence began to fail, and this was compounded by the budding sexuality that my mother did not teach me to manipulate. Sometimes I wonder if it would have helped if I had learned earlier that my body was something to disguise. That might have prepared me better for what was to come.

From inside the house, I could hear the thwack of my brother's basketball against pavement and backboard, a mesmerizing sound, rhythmic yet irregular as my own breath. Mom wasn't home yet, and I felt at a loss, tranquil in the zone of still air provided by the house yet irritable with the way I felt my cells rubbing against each other. Though the squeak of Kelly's tennis shoes and the slap of the ball seemed far, far off, they bounced incessantly between my ears.

My head hurt and my body ached. I had become so pasty and wasted that my brother had taken to calling me "Flat-Bottom Boat." Awkwardly I maneuvered around the house, poling my way with crutches, a cast still on the ankle I'd broken a few weeks before when I fell from my horse. Taut skin over skeleton, I floated, bumped into doorframes and furniture, a clumsy and pointed canoe indeed, and looked for something I would have the energy to do.

I docked myself on the floor in the living room, paging through a magazine without reading, watching the weak winter sun flicker through the limbs of the trees in the backyard, eating Hershey's Kisses out of the turquoise glass candy jar on the coffee table. Holding and twirling the transparent candy-jar lid in front of my eyes, I thought about the spatial division—sofa, lamp, hefty armchair all out there, me under watery glass, drowning peacefully. I peeled another Kiss and balled the foil, almost wanting to bite it, to make of it a filling in my perfect teeth that had felt so funny lately, to chew and swallow something that might make me feel full with its substance. Even the pale winter sunlight felt good on my skin, and I drowsed, cheek to the carpet, the residue of chocolate a comforting thickness in my mouth.

Vaguely, I was aware that I was not well, but I didn't care. I was too tired. I was too sleepy. My cast was too heavy.

Out of that remote world where there was still noise, however, the telephone rang, and I raised myself slow as molasses to answer it. A crisp female voice asked for my mother, and I replied that she was not home yet. "Could I take a message?" I asked in the polite manner of the well-trained child. "No, no," she said, "but tell her to call Dr. Verner's office immediately."

A tube of blood had been drawn painfully from my arm at Dr. Verner's office a few days before, and I paused as I hung up the phone because now I knew clearly that I was ill. The nurse wouldn't tell me the results of the test, even though she knew that I was the one tested. She had not told me that everything would be all right. This had to mean the results were bad. Even in my weary, fuzzy state, I could figure that out.

My mother had already proffered a suspected diagnosis. Because I had been in a wheelchair for six weeks, with broken finger and ankle, and only just recently promoted to crutches, my condition had made itself obvious. Washing my hair, dressing me, helping me to the bathroom, my mother felt under her helpful hands my limbs shrivel like stalks of drought-dry grass. She fetched endless glasses of iced tea and saw that nothing slaked my thirst. It seemed unbelievable that yet another physical calamity should befall me, but she remembered from childhood a Cherry Ames nurse story about the unmistakable symptoms of diabetes: weight loss, excessive thirst, frequent urination, fruity breath.

"You smelled," she would ever after recall, "like an overripe banana."

Only the weekend before, spending the night with friends of the family, I had impressed everyone by peeing every fifteen minutes. I had sat with Sharon and Stacy, playing Parchesi, eating chips and drinking Coke, while their father watched TV and their mother hovered. The lines on her face deepened every time I scrambled up to go to the bathroom. I hardly slept all night, afraid I would wet the bed. No one else slept much either, as I had clomped up and down the hall, announcing the urgency of my overworked bladder each time. When my mother picked me up the next morning, she and Mrs. Fortner exchanged whispers out by the car. Speaking hastily across the open car door, both of them glanced toward the porch where we girls made one last set of cat's cradles in the strings looped around our fingers. Our mothers' eyes struck me over and over with cold worry, and I felt tingling darts along my bare wrists. Only later would I know that this sensation was probably a nerve reaction to my elevated blood sugar.

At the time, I only knew that the looks that people gave me had changed over the past two months. From approving smiles beaming back into my pink-cheeked face and fond pats on my platinum-crowned head, responses of relatives, teachers, friends, and strangers had all become frowning and grim, pitying and repulsed, simultaneously judgmental and bland. I knew I didn't look good, but the broken bones were supposed to be a temporary condition, so I hadn't thought much about it. Now something crept over me, forcing my eyes across the bony wrists sticking from my coat sleeves, showing me the red rubbed marks from the crutch handles, making me stare down at the grotesque knobs of my knees.

This feeling, and the evolution of the glances I earned, slid through my mind when the nurse called, and I hobbled back into the living room and resumed eating Hershey's Kisses, understanding crudely, thinking that perhaps this would be the last time I would have a chance to savor chocolate. The truth was that I would taste chocolate again, but that the easy sense of an appreciative universe would be gone forever. I would miss that far more than any sweets.

Anyway, although I knew I shouldn't be eating the candy, I was ravenously hungry, and afraid. Under my jeans, my hipbones jutted up like beware-of-dog signs and my stomach emitted growls as if the cage of a slavering Doberman. I could see myself reflected in the sliding-glass door, the gray trunks of January trees forming a skeletal backdrop outside. I felt as skinny and wooden as they, and I raised one crutch over my head in imitation of the reaching branches. Finally, I plopped into the rocking chair, looking between my reflection and my actual body. In the glass, my heavy, brown, octagonal-shaped eyeglasses overwhelmed my pale face, and my hair hung dull and stringy all around. But worse were the surfaces and sensations of my body up close. My right ring finger, crooked and scarred from being broken, pierced laterally with a traction pin, and then growing to the foam rubber padding of the splint, refused to fold neatly into place next to my other fingers. Texture-wise, the surface of my skin had become peculiar—dry and almost stiff with dehydration, but oily to the point of slime in patches over my face and torso. Unless something was in my mouth, causing my saliva to flow, it dried up like poured concrete, my tongue stuck like a footprint in an old sidewalk. My left arm sported an oblong green bruise from the blood sugar test of a few days before, and I could not forget the sensation of that long needle sliding into my arm so purposefully.

The afternoon shadows lengthened, I listened to the outside—boys playing basketball, cars swishing down the street, dogs barking in the twilight—and felt my own lassitude. That world receded further and further as I drifted into a different kind of awareness. Around me the house stood, a protection, a box, a prison, a haven, a moat, an almost inescapable divider. The house became my body, and my body only a dysfunctional part. I imagined that I was some internal organ my mom had called a pancreas and that I could no longer do anything inside this body of a house but instead lay passive, inert. I thought of the texture of severed chicken livers, dense and glistening—they were all I knew of internal organs.

For a moment my mind reached toward a book, roamed the back rooms, even ran into the barn and pasture across the street. So much waited for me. I still wanted to do things! Then even the living room retreated, and I realized that I was inside, not only inside the house, but looking and experiencing inside my body, not only the surface in the glass reflection, but further inside, in the land of long veins like rubber bands, of stringy intestines and soupy cavities, where food was transformed into something entirely different from itself, properly or not. Everyone else was still outside; I had this space all to myself.

It was, if not a pretty place to be, an interesting one. The rhythms of my heart and my breathing comforted me in a peaceful dual pattern of systole and diastole, in and out, rise and fall, one and two. My ribs protectively hugged my lungs, my breasts seemed to be growing as a cushion for my heart. I had always flushed easily, and, now, when the hyped-up metabolism of uncontrolled diabetes combined with the slightest embarrassment or exertion, I could literally feel the blood flow into my face, the capillaries expand and open, the heat come to the surface of my skin so hard and fast that it sometimes felt as if there were no blood left in my heart and major arteries. I could also, for some reason, feel my huge, hidden eyeballs in my head and, when I closed my eyes, see the image of blood vessels, little snakes of vision stretching toward the light. Certainly I could feel the hollow bag of my stomach, the pain of its emptiness outlining its shape and size as clearly as any metal pointer during an autopsy for medical students.

In this, my first experience of the inwardness of illness, of a future of defining myself from internal states, I realized that I'd at least partially lost contact with what was external to me, even my own appearance and demeanor. I did not analyze the feelings, but, though I could see that my cuteness had withered, I did not want to connect to the fearful glances people had started giving me—they had to be looking at something or someone else. Granted, too, that perhaps my internal and external states were pretty well matched that day, but soon enough that too was untrue. I had to develop the ability to pay attention to a whole range of physical phenomena that others could not even see, and this focus meant that other information—from the surface—was blocked.

Over the years, other people have marveled at how well I know my body. Because I constantly monitor myself—signs of low and high blood sugar and all the related minor "symptoms" of complications—it seems to others that I am unusually in touch with my own physicality. And I am. Internally. But the outside? My skin, the contours of my face, the proportions of my legs, the shapes of my breasts, belly, ass—my connections to the rest of the world? Even standing naked in front of a full-length mirror, I still cannot see them clearly.

But I always retained the desire to please, and so I paid ever closer attention to others' faces in response to my appearance. I have read those faces as though they were mirrors, as though I could see myself only through them. I think I am searching these faces for clues about my fate, based on a moment in time when nobody told me very much. That day early in 1972, I waited for what seemed like a long time before my mother came home. When she arrived and called the doctor's office, her face knit itself into a web of pained wrinkles and grieved furrows. She put her hand tenderly on my cheek, and looked at me with fear and horror.

To this day, whenever someone frowns, I have a tendency to feel ugly, sometimes even sick, all over again.

The results of that first blood sugar test defined me most certainly as having diabetes mellitus, "juvenile," as they called it then, with a ratio of more than 400 mg/dl (milligrams per deciliter) of glucose in my blood. I was not far from ketoacidosis and coma. Her face set with grim determination, my mother packed me a suitcase and loaded me up in the car for another ride to the hospital. But this time things were different. No longer a knock-about kid with a couple of broken bones, waiting in the gruesomely fascinating hubbub of a crowded emergency room, I was this time ushered quietly through carpeted halls, and not into the children's ward because it was full, but into a large, empty room on a silent, tense floor.

What I remember most about that stay in the hospital is needles. My thin arms soon enough were tracked up and down with bruises and punctures, as in those days a full tube of blood was needed just to determine the moment's blood sugar. Ah, for the quick finger-prick technology of today, but it didn't exist then. Soon, it was discovered that I was cursed with "rolling" veins, so that most samples required that the needle be turned and gouged back and forth, as the lucky seeker sought to catch the vein as it turned evasively in my arm. I dreaded the arrival of the technicians and when one mistakenly told me that I would be "giving blood" every hour all night I wept uncontrollably until a nurse asked me what was wrong. Hysterical, I could hardly tell her, but soon enough she corrected the error and left me lying in a barren pool of white light in the dark room, relieved, but drained, staring at a wall that I did not see.

With that I had overstepped my allotment of tears, and I did not cry about my diabetes again in front of people. Instead, I focused on my arms as morbid attractions, their swirls of earthy colors like watercolor landscapes and the pattern of punctures like clock faces plotting out important moments of the future and past. I was fascinated at how the blood could leak under the skin, how the body eventually cleaned up and repaired each little mess, the bruises and pinpricks shifting and fading like each day's sunset. The skin was such a transparent layer, flaking off and replacing itself over and over, and I was nothing but these separate and temporary parts, smelly substances, decaying flesh.

Why, I wondered, did the bruises go away and yet the moles stayed? I fixated on the more permanent status of my moles, especially on my left arm. I spent hours staring and memorizing the patterns, again using the clock face image to make this possible. There were four main clocks: 2:25 near my elbow, 5:49:47 largest and in the middle, 5:10 just below that, and 8:12 just behind my wrist. I was obsessed with the idea that my mother should also memorize these patterns, in case I should disappear and a replica or substitute of some sort should masquerade as me. Surely no one, no matter how diabolical, would have the ability to duplicate me down to the moles on my arm. I never, in all the years I had this fantasy, thought about whether or not my replacement would have diabetes.

Would anyone recognize me through all the physical changes? No longer cute, I searched for other ways to assure myself this was actually my own body. Somehow, I wanted affirmation that someone knew me, understood the essence of me, would miss me if I were gone. What I got was a lot of attention to the practical matters of keeping me around, but little acknowledgment of the painfulness of what I knew: that I had a serious illness that would almost certainly shorten my life and which could arbitrarily end it at any time. Although improvements in treatment since then have rendered differences in life expectancy minimal for those of us in good control, the diagnosis had altered every thread of my existence.

About the fourth day of my stay, my mother returned from her first and only meeting of the American Diabetes Association support group. "You're not leaving the hospital until you can give yourself your own shot," she said, wearing the dogged, stubborn expression that was becoming so frequent on her face. She had found the meeting full of whining self-pity, and the contents of her stomach rose dangerously as she listened to a mother of a teenage girl who still refused to give herself injections. Whenever the girl wanted to attend a sleepover, her mother would get up and drive across town to the friend's home in the morning to administer her shot.

"You have to be able to take care of yourself," my mom said, and I nodded my agreement. Just like with the braids, I thought. No big deal.

Doing it was another thing. Injecting sterile water into oranges proved fun, and I played for hours, my boredom relieved slightly, the bright color and soft shape of the fruit welcome in the dull, white room with its square, sterile surfaces. But I would hunch for hours over my thigh, my left hand urging the scarce flesh into a dimpled mound, the syringe posed spearlike in my right hand, unable to stab. Self-mutilation would never have been my choice, but here I was, learning it in the hospital. Everything in me resisted. I didn't want to hurt myself. I held my arms a hundred different ways, varying angle, height, distance from my sides. I tried closing my eyes, but could still sense when the needle drew near my skin. I tried to force myself into the quick, casual motion that was so easy with the orange. Nope. Nothing doing. So, against the nurses' teaching, I tried a slow approach, resting the tip of the needle on my leg and trying to talk myself into pushing it in. I could bear the pain of the very tip of the needle in my skin, I found, but to shove it into the firm flesh was more than I could bear.

Besides, hadn't I done enough already? In spite of its repugnance, I had mastered the skill of urine testing right away. Every time I peed, I caught some in a clear plastic cup. Then I opened a little kit in a vertical stand, opened and dropped a Clinitest tablet into the test tube, took the eyedropper and measured out three golden tears of stinky pee into the tube, and waited to see it bubble and change into malevolent colors that I had to compare to a chart to see how much sugar was there. In the hospital, I thought, this is okay, but in the bathroom at school, no way. The entire setup had to be washed and laid out to dry every time, and I began to imagine that my fingers, even scrubbed with soap and disinfectant, reeked of urine. Eventually, the urine tests would become more of a problem than the shots, but at first it seemed almost natural in comparison to sticking needles in my body.

Once, at age five, I had stepped on a nail, instantly bending and pulling it out, as my toe bled into the grass in the backyard.

That whole sense of something alien invading one's body—it was worse than the pain! But the nail had been an accidental collision; now I was being asked to do this intentionally. The space is already occupied by me, I thought, how can something else be forced into that same space? It was too weird that we weren't solid after all, but permeable, insubstantial, wobbly. How could I ever again feel the same about the surface of my body?

A few days earlier, I'd sat in the living room, looking into an inner self ever divided from the world; now I saw that the world was not so separate, that I was subject to its incursions at any time. And worse, neither idea canceled the other out, the paradox being the most horrible truth of them both. Isolation and vulnerability to invasion, both delivered via the same little syringe.

For days I had disappointed my keepers. Every nurse on the floor, at every shift during the day, had tried her hand at encouraging me. We had all failed together, and patience was growing short, even among those who used the gentle approach. The days had been an Everywoman parade, as various nurses represented a panoply of psychological strategies to get me to stick the needle in my leg. There was the Fun Approach—see? your leg is just like the orange, see how fast you can jab it. There was the Tough Approach—no big deal, just do it. And there was the Sympathetic Approach—I'm so sorry, but it has to be done. In all of them there was the idea that I should be a brave girl. "Make it easier on everyone," one of the nurses finally sighed in exasperation, glancing guiltily over her shoulder to make sure no one else heard, "and don't be such a fraidy-cat."

The nurses on my floor, after all, did not usually deal with children, and I never saw or heard another kid while I was in the hospital. Only a monotonous roar of televisions, P.A. system bells and pages, and whispered conversation floated in my door, and I seldom left the room. At night, I might be awakened by the moans, sometimes shouts, of the man across the hall, and I dreaded it, but in the morning it seemed like a dream. For me, stuck in this odd ward full of older patients, there was no one to play cards with in the long hours of the day, no one with whom to compare injuries and symptoms, no cheerfully decorated playroom or lobby, no camaraderie. I met no diabetics who could give themselves shots and no other youngsters who had learned difficult treatment regimens. Of course, I resisted.

Eventually, the task was accomplished with the clever help of a candy striper. I still remember her with all the awe and fondness accorded a savior, her bright face and her helpful lies. As part of the encouraging entourage, she had visited me at least once during each of her shifts, always popping her head politely in the door, her eyebrows raised cheerfully and expectantly in a question of whether I had done it yet. She exuded an unusual sincerity, as though she thought it really was her job to help people. A few years later, when I was fourteen, I followed her example and became a candy striper myself, but, ironically, the hospital considered me too young to work with patients and assigned me to work at the gift shop, the main feature of which was a huge selection of fresh candy displayed old-style in glass jars and scooped and weighed into individual bags by me. I bought and ate tons of it on the sly, and quit after a few months, feeling as though I had helped no one. I've often wondered if my candy striper knew how much she helped me, even had the notion of going on *Unsolved Mysteries* to see if I could locate and thank her, though it probably wouldn't merit a segment because she didn't do anything as dramatic as pull me from a burning or sinking-in-the-water car.

What she did was to cut a deal with me: she'd let me try it on her first if I'd go on and do it to myself immediately afterward. She said she wasn't afraid because it wouldn't hurt anyway. If I had to do it the rest of my life, she said, she could certainly let me try it on her once.

To shoot her in the arm with the ubiquitous sterile water, I sat Indian-legged on the bed, facing her side. She sat firmly on the edge of the bed, looking out the window at the gray February sky and the ugly roof of the neighboring wing of the building, a professional smile fixed on her face. Around us fanned an audience of the concerned: my parents, a floor nurse, all the witnesses necessary to test me, to urge me on, to sigh again if I failed.

Hands cold and with a show of false bravado, I expertly filled the syringe and tapped out the bubbles. This was something I could do, but I knew that it meant nothing, that the hard part remained. The candy striper's pushed-up sleeve revealed a smooth, tanned bicep, which I took reluctantly between my blue-white fingers, first pinching up too much flesh, then too little, adjusting the pressure to the resistance I could feel growing in her muscle tissue, which quivered in spite of her posture, straight and stalwart as a tongue depressor.

The airy dart-throw technique still evaded me, and finally I braced the side of my right hand against her warm skin and with small jerks planted the needle bit by bit into her arm. This seemed to take forever, my peripheral vision going dim, a rivulet of sweat running frightened down my back, and midway she sucked the air in through her teeth and tensed her arm in spite of herself. I knew I was hurting her, and as soon as I could I pulled the syringe back out of her flesh. Then I recoiled. Where I had squeezed with my left hand, I could see the scarlet imprints of my fingers. Where I had withdrawn the needle, a purple-green bruise already swelled around the nimbus of the tiny but angry puncture wound.

Everyone in the room breathed together in a heaving sigh of relief instead of one of disappointment. "Now, see? That was easy," the young woman said. "Piece of cake." I smiled at the metaphor, but no one else seemed to notice, focused as they were on cheering me on to injecting myself.

After that, my own leg seemed fairly easy to stick with a needle, but I must admit that I've never really mastered the technique of the quick and painless jab. Certainly, the less I'm thinking about it the better it is, and most of the time it really doesn't hurt much, as the needles have shrunk to a filament thinness, but always I remain aware of the crossing of the boundary of my body. Taking shots is the least of my troubles as a diabetic— almost nothing—except when I pause and think about the permeable surface of my skin, my being.

In December, I'd had a traction pin drilled through the end of my right ring finger, and the doctor had only a few days before pulled it out with a pair of pliers. I had been afraid that with it gone I'd be able to see through the hole, from one side of my finger out the other, but instead blood trickled out each side and the finger's solidity reasserted itself. Giving shots is similarly strange, and even now when shooting up, I often think about painter Frida Kahlo, impaled on a pole in a girlhood tram accident, about the dagger entering the breast of Juliet with a stab she suddenly finds is different from that of love, about the bayonets of World War I, the shrapnel of World War II, the machine-gun fire of Korea and Vietnam, transforming living bodies into meat. It's not the pain that bothers me, but the creepy violence of other matter merging with mine.

At eleven, I wasn't ready for this idea, much less for its physical fact. And yet, as with so much of growing up (or refusing to), something happens and you either face it or you don't. We are called upon, so to speak, both happily (as in falling in love, receiving a scholarship or job offer in some new and far-off place, or embarking on writing a book) and unhappily (in the face of illness, death, and other types of loss and trauma). We have little choice about when these things happen in life, but we do choose whether to grow or shrivel.

I'm grateful that I was able, with that young woman's help, to take the first big step toward growing up. Sitting on the hospital bed, with an expectant audience, I performed. In earning others' relief and approval, I learned that doing for others often is also doing for oneself. Alongside that, however, I encountered my own solitary nature in the heavy responsibility that would never leave me, not for a waking or sleeping instant, though I might rail and rage and plead and despair over it. Staring down at my leg, taking the plunge, swallowing my fear of my body, I learned that I was so much more than just that mass of flesh.

I was also beginning to understand that others seldom really feel this way, no matter their rhetoric, that people's attitudes about me differ once they know the truth about my body. Our society has an elaborate system of denial in the face of our biology, and suddenly the Emperor's clothes were stripped away. I could see him, and myself, naked, but no one else seemed to notice.

During the elevator ride up to my room the night I'd been admitted to the hospital, my family stood hushed and somber, as I leaned tiredly against the wall with my crutches. Facing us, and our obvious distress over what seemed to her a minor event, a nurse patted my cheek, pointed at my cast, and said, "That'll be all healed in no time, don't you worry," before cheerily exiting the elevator and leaving us further stunned and embarrassed.

This misapprehension of my illness soon became a theme, and has remained so all these years. When you have a disease that no one can see, you are alone with it in a peculiar way: the more obviously ill and handicapped may be rejected out of hand, but with diabetes you are accepted, to the extent that you can "pass." And, I might emphasize, *only* so far as you seem "normal." What this creates is a division of self, the "abnormal" hidden within the "normal," the body primed to betray its secrets, the rejections delayed but looming. I have learned over the years to expect them, and many friends have commented on this trait of skittish anticipation of the worst. This attitude, however strange and sad it seems, reflects my reality. I am always a guest in the good graces of others, and, directly or indirectly, it is my body that will turn them away from me.

This lesson began to take root in my mind immediately, and budding adolescent femaleness soon reinforced it. A few short weeks after my diagnosis, my broken ankle was deemed healed and the cast was removed from my leg, an oddly shrunken limb that no longer seemed mine. The muscle was stringy and wasted, dead skin in chalky layers flaked from my surface, and long black hairs the likes of which I'd never seen emerged through the powdery crud like strange weeds, prickly as burrs, sharp as scissorgrass. Home from the doctor's office, I locked myself in the bathroom, scrubbed until my skin turned red, and shaved until the razor was packed with detritus. Already I had a typical horror of the real, mature female body. In another few weeks, the first brown stains appeared on my underwear, another phenomenon to hide at all costs. I developed a horror of and disbelief in the tampon commercials that depicted slim young girls in white pants. Never, never would I wear such clothing. They could keep the white pants in the same dustbin as the girdles, the one as overly revealing as the other was oppressive. Soon, my skin was breaking out from scalp to waist, and within months, I began gaining significant amounts of weight and metamorphosed from skinny to plump. I no longer knew myself.

And so, I did what we all do. I covered myself and I hid what all women hide—menstruation, bulges, hair, pimples—and the extra mess of urine tests and injection sites. The women that I wanted to be like were smooth, nice-smelling, and functioned as imperceptibly as the grass grew. I took to wearing high collars and long pants in dark colors, continued to let my hair grow as a veil over my ears, neck, and face, and took to filthy bathroom stalls to take my shots. No one wanted to see the truth, and I wasn't about to make them. Although in the back of my head I wanted to believe there were more important things than cosmetic beauty, I thought the truth was just as gross as most people did. It was just that because of my diabetes I knew that the ugly truth was me.

2

Good Enough

Two over-easy eggs steamed and stared up at me from the glassy surface of the plate, yolk leaking from one like a yellow tear and the crusty edge of the other curled into a greasy frown. The three pieces of whole-wheat toast already seemed to scratch and claw their way down my throat, the pulp of the orange juice tied itself around my teeth, and my mucus thickened into a glob around my glottis in anticipation of the tall glass of milk. I felt sick. In the weeks after my diagnosis with diabetes, breakfast had become an ordeal.

Dr. Hawkes, the highly recommended specialist who had become my doctor, believed in breakfast. All I remember about her was her iron-gray hair and her fanatical diatribe about the importance of the first meal of the day. Almost like the highest form of faith and morality, eating a good breakfast was a requirement of her care, especially when one had wasted away, as I had, into skeletal form from weeks of uncontrolled diabetes, excreting all unused sugars and living off fat and muscle, the body breaking itself down because it cannot take hold of food. In those days, virtually no one practiced patient-centered medicine. What you were given was a prescription: do this, no protests please.

My family habitually had partaken of what Dr. Hawkes indicated were weak, corrupt breakfasts. We always ate in the morning, but usually we quickly downed a bowl of cereal and a small glass of juice, just enough to get the U.S. RDA of vitamin C. Although not guilty of the Pop-Tart sin, horror of horrors, we sometimes resorted to Carnation Instant Breakfast. We were duly chastised, but I continued to have trouble with the change. That much food in the morning grossed me out.

Unfortunately, it never occurred to any of us to question Dr. Hawkes's directions. Because I was so thin, Dr. Hawkes said I needed to gain weight quickly. I had grown tall as the proverbial weed during the past year and was well over the average for my age—almost five feet five already—but instead of gaining a concomitant amount of weight, I had lost nearly ten pounds in the past few months and didn't even bounce the scale to ninety pounds, including the weight of the heavy cast on my leg. My bony hands, with large knuckles protruding through my withered skin, revealed the strength and substance of a robust bone structure, now abandoned by flesh. My weight would have stabilized on its own eventually had I eaten a normal amount of food, but Dr. Hawkes put me on a 3,000-calorie diet. Nowadays this sounds incredible, and it's hard to imagine anyone prescribing or trying to follow such a plan, but back then we thought that doctors knew best. I would sit at the table, meal after meal, choking down the assigned number of calories. Of course, by the time I reached thirteen, my girth had widened too far. Now we know that excess insulin in our system (whether due to injection or to Type 2 diabetes, where insulin is present but underutilized) makes it very difficult for diabetics to control our weight. The last thing in the world I needed was to be taught to overeat. But that is precisely what, in accord with that era's protocol, Dr. Hawkes recommended I do.

By the time I was fifteen and weighing in at over 150, I hated her for it. Once I had gotten my strength back, I would never again obey a doctor without question.

When I was thirteen, we moved back from big-city Memphis to small-city Knoxville, which boasted no diabetic specialists. First, we went to an allergist recommended by Dr. Hawkes, but within a couple of visits it became clear that he knew nothing about diabetes and was merely a med school buddy of hers. An old man with an unsympathetic style, he was completely uninterested in and at a loss to deal with the issues of my weight, my severe menstrual cramps, and the blood sugar difficulties posed by the unpredictable world of high school. He asked the same questions over and over again at our first appointment, as if trying to catch me out in a lie or an inconsistency, or as if he simply could not comprehend my answers. Menstrual cramps, he said, were just something I'd have to learn to bear. Docile as we were, after a couple of visits my mother and I had had enough.

We switched to a young internist who had treated my grandmother in the nursing home, as my mom had been impressed by his laid-back manner and his diagnosis of my grandmother's sodium deficiency. Perhaps he would be more responsive since he was younger. True, Dr. Gilbertson's hair showed only a sprinkle of gray and his big, blue eyes were fringed with long, flirtatious lashes. He was young, but, unfortunately, his patients were mostly elderly.

In the waiting room, I was a complete oddity, eyed by the bleared and ailing ancient. I could almost hear them thinking, "What the hell is she doing here?" and I more than once wondered this myself. Copies of *Modern Maturity* and *Sunset* littered the lobby, 85-degree air blasted from the vents, and the nurses came to the door shouting people's names into the room, which except for the occasional clack of shifting dentures and a few labored sighs, was silent. These old people all seemed cowed and afraid, trembling their way to the inner office on canes and walkers, glancing beseechingly up at crisp nurses, their worn and wrinkled clothes in sharp contrast to the professional glare of white uniforms. Usually we waited two hours past our appointment time, and I spent the hours imagining what these people had been like at my age. When called by a nurse, I stood as tall as possible, looked her right in the face, and strode with enough pride for everyone in the room.

They must have hated to see me coming, not only because I flounced, nor mainly because my urine-sugar test records could always have been better, but for two other reasons: my veins didn't like to give up their blood and, truly, the staff had little to offer in the way of treatment advice. All of the advances in diabetes treatment made possible by home blood sugar testing simply weren't available then. Doctors were proscriptive because they were helpless otherwise.

My treatment consisted of one daily injection of an insulin suspension designed to deliver peaks three times a day, one to "cover" each meal. Keeping the peaks of the insulin's action and the sugar load from food in line with each other necessitated a strict time routine: I had to take my shot and eat my meals at exactly the same times every day, or I'd be in trouble. Exercise, which like insulin lowers blood sugar, ideally needed to be consistent as well. And, to make sure that other influences—illness, "cheating," emotional ups and downs, variations in activity, gradual changes in the course of the disease—weren't affecting my blood sugar too much, I peed in a plastic cup and tested my urine for sugar, ideally four times a day, before each meal and at bedtime.

At Dr. Gilbertson's, once every few months, the nurse would draw a tube of blood and test it for an actual blood glucose reading. There was no discussion of how I'd been feeling, what changes in routine or activity I might be dealing with, whether my appetite and weight were stable, how many insulin reactions I'd had, whether I'd had infections or other signs of high blood sugar, or any other aspect of this complicated, life-saturating condition. Once the test result was ready, I would sit across the desk in Dr. Gilbertson's huge, dim office, and he would bestow on me a harangue about how I needed to do better with my urine tests. That was all.

Once I tried to tell him that the lower urine-test results he wanted made me feel terrible, but he waved his hand, narrowed his baby blues, and told me to quit making excuses. In an instant shock, I recognized that he would never believe a word I said. What he cared about were the numbers—urine tests and the blood glucose test I would have each office visit, though such a reading once every three months tells you less than a parole meeting with an ex-con because blood sugar can change rapidly and frequently.

Today, diabetics test their blood sugars at home—I do so as often as six times a day—and once every few months we have a glycosylated hemoglobin test, which gives an approximate blood sugar average for a several-week period of time. In 1975, all a good blood sugar test meant was that you hadn't skipped any injections or eaten any candy bars in the couple of days before you went to the doctor. What it measured in any particular moment told you next to nothing about the overall control of a person's diabetes. Still, scant as it was, it was all we had in the way of information.

Except for the urine tests that I did at home. This was the only test available to help you see on a daily basis how the insulin you were taking by injection every day was matched to the food you were digesting. But urine sugar measures were crude at best, with only five intervals (negative, +1, +2, +3, and +4) covering the span of possible blood sugars from 0 mg/dl, where you would be dead of hypoglycemia, to the 1,000 mg/dl or so that would mean ketoacidosis, coma, and death from elevated blood sugar. "Negative" made no distinction between normal and too low, and when I kept my urine sugars at the lower end of the scale I would continually suffer episodes of low blood sugar.

These could happen anywhere and anytime—on the school bus on the way home, on horseback out in the fields, in my room as I played alone or did my homework, at the mall as I shopped with my friends, or in bed at night as I slept unaware. Most of the time, I would begin to shake, my hands fumbling to button my coat, my legs growing loose around the pony, my handwriting spiraling incoherent across the page, my feet dragging a little as I walked. I might realize that I was sweating, or my heart was beating too fast, or that I couldn't do the simplest thing. Then I would pop a few Lifesavers and be back to normal in a few minutes, though sometimes exhausted, a ring of confusion remaining around my head until I'd had a good night's sleep.

But sometimes low blood sugar crept up on me, or I became mean or sad instead of shaky. One cold day when I was fourteen, the school bus dropped my brother and me off at the bottom of the long hill on which we lived, and we began our usual trudge up the steep slope to the house. In a flash, however, I sat down on the pavement and told my brother I was too tired, that I'd come home in a few minutes. Well coached, he knew that I was wrong and coaxed me on up to the house. I went straight into my bedroom and shut the door.

"Don't you want some juice?" Kelly asked from outside, pushing the door open.

I had flopped backward onto the bed, my coat still on, my gloves still on, my glasses twisted precariously. "Nope. I'm fine," I answered. "Leave me alone."

Fortunately, he did not, but came back instead with a tall glass of juice and several cookies. I was completely annoyed, but he insisted that I drink and eat.

"I knew," he later said, "because your eyes were like glass marbles in your head. No expression whatsoever. You just weren't really there." Certainly, I could hardly remember the incident, and this was horrifying. There I was, walking around, talking, moving, and not seeing anything. It was like being inhabited by an alien from outer space.

Hypoglycemia often happens like this, suddenly and unexpectedly, with no apparent variation from the usual routine, and the drop from the normal blood glucose of 80 mg/dl to zero is not far. Unconsciousness and death can happen in a matter of minutes or hours, rather than the days and weeks it takes for high blood sugar to kill you. And a low blood sugar can make you irrational, so that you ignore symptoms and fail to treat yourself, appearing drunk or crazy instead of ill before you pass out. It is responsible for 32,000 emergency diabetic hospitalizations a year.

The first such hypoglycemic hospitalization for me occurred when I was fourteen and did not get up one Sunday morning, although my father had made his special pancakes and had the sugar-free syrup out on the table. In my bedroom downstairs, I had not responded to his call from the top of the stairs. When he came to the door, irritated at my ignoring him, he could see me lying there, staring at him from under the covers, my eyes blank to the point of malevolence. I would not answer him, and he stalked back upstairs where my mother was putting the plates out on the kitchen counter.

"She's ignoring me," my father said, waving the spatula in the air. He thought that I was being some kind of brat. But in the next moment, he and my mother both realized what was happening.

"She's having a reaction," my mother said, reaching for the orange juice and a glass, both of them heading for the stairs.

When I came to, my mother was pouring juice down my throat, my father hovered with the spatula still in hand, and my head was suffused with one long, sharp, and undulating pain. Immediately, I began to vomit all over the bed and then passed out from the pain into a deep blackness. Between bouts of agonized wakefulness, in which the pain seemed unbearable and the retching worse, and peaceful moments of unconsciousness, I began to understand the situation. My mother held my head and guided my further heaves into the plastic trash can from the bathroom; my father, on the telephone in the next room, received instructions to take me to the emergency room. They bundled me into bathrobe and blanket, and I crawled into the backseat of the car and lay down, as if I could hide from the sunlight, the motion, the intense throbbing in my temples and the wringing of my now-empty intestines. The main thing that registered was the speed with which my father drove, and I clutched the edge of the seat with a dim, terrifying sensation of the centrifugal force sliding me against the door. I wondered briefly if it was locked, then conked out again.

I don't remember much of anything until I was wakened several hours later, still in the emergency room, after I'd been treated with nausea and pain medications and allowed to sleep. According to the nurse who wakened me, I was ready to go home, but I told her I couldn't get up, that it would make me sick again. I begged for her to let me lie there and sleep some more, but she coaxed and prodded me toward the wheelchair, behind which my father stood ready to roll me out. As soon as I sat up, I puked again. They admitted me to the hospital that night, and by morning I felt better, though I wondered why no one ever seemed to believe me when it came to my disease.

We did not receive any explanation for this extreme version of insulin shock. Was the pain a migraine, like the ones my brother sometimes suffered? The doctors called it a migraine, but didn't want to speculate on family patterns. Was the migraine caused by low blood sugar, or vice versa? They couldn't tell. How likely was this sort of thing to happen again? No one said, but I knew I wanted to avoid it.

Thus I developed my sense of the fine balance between high and low that is of utmost importance, this high-wire act that requires constant tuning and adjustment. Years of exposure to elevated blood glucose damages the body's tissues—especially the heart, kidneys, nerves, and blood vessels in the eyes and extremities—and causes premature but gradual death to most diabetics. And outright diabetic ketoacidosis (resulting from high blood sugar) still kills far more diabetics (about 1,750 a year), usually before they are diagnosed or because some other illness has disrupted their ability to treat the disease. But it is hypoglycemia that can kill you on any given day when you least expect it and so hangs like a cleaver in your consciousness.

When Dr. Gilbertson admonished me to keep my urine tests lower, I would nod, knowing full well that I would not. His advice was doubtless by the book, but it conflicted with what kept me feeling well. Only after I had had diabetes ten years, when after college I finally visited a specialist in Minneapolis, did a doctor tell me that I must have had what was called a low renal threshold; that it didn't take much sugar in my blood for it to reach my urine. "They should have told you to shoot for plus two, instead of negative or plus one," she said. But they hadn't.

Rather, I figured out on my own that I needed to keep on doing things my way. Too much was at stake for me not to. Going to the doctor became an ordeal I endured every few months, but it had nothing to do with my daily life. It was an empty ritual, and the care of my diabetes became essentially my own.

Having given up the idea of doing what the doctors dictated, I nonetheless still silently suffered their ministrations at their offices. We all pretended that the ordeal was worth the trouble, though I didn't really believe it. I remember one occasion in particular, when the nurse couldn't manage to get the blood out of my thin, rolling, collapsible veins.

She was new, pert and pretty, and reeked of inexperience, but I resigned myself to her cheeriness and let her seat me in the chair with the shelf snapping into place in front of me. I always hated the feeling of being trapped in these seats. I mean, who were they kidding that they had to lock you in so that you'd have something to prop your arm on? They just didn't want you to be able to flee. Such were the thoughts coursing through my head as the nurse pushed up my sleeves and pulled my turned-up arms out in front of me for her perusal.

"The left one is usually best," I said, pulling my right hand out of her grasp and pointing. "There's a pretty good one right up there."

Her eyes darkened slightly. "I think I prefer this one," she said, regaining my right arm and indicating a vague green smudge right in the crease of my elbow. Oh well, I thought, I can carry my books on my left arm for a few days.

After she had tied the tourniquet around my arm, I turned my head away and tried to focus on the milky white of the enameled cabinets. "Can't you bear to watch it?" the nurse asked, thumping on the submerged vein and turning my arm side to side.

"I always jerk a little bit if I watch," I answered, "and that's no fun for anyone."

She jabbed. And missed. I turned to look as she pulled back on the plunger and got nothing. Quickly, she pulled the needle out. "You're right," she smiled stiffly. "Let's try that other one."

The second and third tries, both on the left arm, and the fourth, back on the right, went on much longer but yielded the same result. Nothing. Try as she might, the nurse could not get the needle to pierce my veins. As my entire body clenched in pain, the nurse moved the needle back and forth under my skin, twisting it sideways to try to nick the vein, turning it this way and that at various depths of penetration. I felt as though a molly bolt had been screwed into my arm.

Eventually, they would send me across the street to the hospital lab, where an old country woman would sit me down, shake her head over the mangled condition of my arms, and tell me to "milk a cow" for her. Within seconds, a tube of dark blood would glitter in her hand like the world's largest ruby. But for an eternity, I sat underneath the shadow of Dr. Gilbertson's nurse as more and more intently she bent over me. I slumped further and further down in the chair, my arms unnaturally upturned like the legs of a splayed roadkill, trying to remember that this was no big deal.

"I can feel it," she gasped out once. "I must've crossed it. All I have to do is pull back a little." But she pulled back too far, and the vein slipped away like an unhooked fish. By now, my eyes were on her face, where the makeup disintegrated like ice on a spring lake and little beads of perspiration hung in her hair like raindrops on tree branches. She made a few more heartless digs before giving up.

"I can't get it," she croaked over her shoulder to one of the other nurses, who patted her on the elbow sympathetically. She backed away from me as though I had tried to shoot her, hands raised, face pale. And, then, as I lay near fainting, she had the nerve to cry.

"It's okay," I whispered. "Really."

I wanted to be a good sport, a great kid, a brave girl, a charming woman. I had grown up, after all, with the tired adage that "pretty is as pretty does," and for a long time—much longer than I denied the fearful mortality of my body's beauty—I tried to live up to that, to believe it. Allure, if it didn't reside in my face, should exude from my personality. But I was like the child who draws a picture on the kitchen wall to please Mommy and Daddy: I could never get on the right wavelength.

It became clearer and clearer that not only my body was a problem, but my temperament was too. My pain was just something else that was ugly, and I found it impossible to maintain the cheerful demeanor I thought would veil my physical flaws. My modicum of physical attractiveness, I grew to believe, would suffice if only I were less eccentric, less demanding, less, well . . . trouble. I was a lot of trouble, and still am, though I never set out to be.

Certainly, some of this lurked in my personality to begin with, and my cussedness and defiance from infancy on are legendary in my family. "You were born," my mother once said, "seven pounds of resistance to the earth." As a baby, I would never lie still, happily burbling in my crib, but wailed unless carried or given a radio for entertainment. I refused to go to sleep unless swaddled and rocked. By the age of five, I stood on the front porch and at a group of loitering high school boys who inadvertently tromped on the flower bed yelled, "Get out of my yard." Posed in a triangle of outrage, my feet apart, hands on my hips, I feared nothing. The boys, the story goes, moved on.

Later, after my broken bones had healed and my diabetes was under control, I fought a pitched battle against the Moneypennys—two older boys from a neighborhood family who liked to break down the pasture fences and chase the horses on their motorbikes. I had tried the niceties, knocking on their door and politely requesting a cease in their trespassing after I had first followed the tracks of their tires from a sagging, unhinged spot in the barbed-wire fence. When that didn't work, and the horses continued to escape into the semi-rural-suburban streets through the holes in the fence, risking traffic accident and death, I devised other strategies. Primary among these was diligence and physical presence. Almost every afternoon after school, I stood, halter or feed bucket as my only protection, between the Moneypennys and the horses. I would chase them out and walk the fence line in the dusk, bolstering the weakened or broken portions so they would hold until the next weekend when my father and I could restring the section. Eventually, it took police threats to their parents—and college—to keep those boys away, but I certainly did my time facing them down.

I try now to love this quality in myself, to admire that girl like a David taking on Goliath, but it's not a characteristic to earn affection in the world. It became, because of my illness, necessary for survival, but it never endeared me to anyone, least of all my family.

When my father, for instance, would say no to some request—Can I have a soda? Can we go to see *Mary Poppins*? Can I spend the night with Sharon and Stacy? Oops. *May* I go to Kim's party Saturday?—I would always come back with "Why not?"

"You would get your way far more often," my mother advised me, "if, instead of being so logical, you would just say 'please.' You know, you catch more flies with honey than with vinegar." What did such recommendations have to do with me, who had to avoid at all costs being sweet? Honey, sugar, sweetie-pie, don't you know that girls are made of sugar and spice and everything nice? Be sweet, be sweet, be sweet. . . . Well, no, I just couldn't.

My father never went along to my doctors' appointments, in fact, never really participated in my care beyond giving me juice when my blood sugar went too low and sometimes making a dinner that fulfilled the requirements. To this day, he has never given me an injection. He credits this to my already-formed personality. "You wouldn't allow me to give you your shot," he recalled when I asked what he remembered about the year of my diagnosis. "You were always so independent and stubborn."

I was stunned by this conversation, because I've considered it one of those signs of familial failure that my father has never in all these years given me a shot. How uninvolved could a parent be? And yet, it came back around to me. I was sure that he was right—it would have been like me to pull away, to reject his attempt to help—but I also found myself angry that the responsibility for everything lay at my feet. I was eleven, after all, and he could have offered again sometime. Our relationship was difficult, however, and mostly we fought and hurt each other's feelings.

Typical of our disagreements was an argument that took place one school night during high school, when a friend called right after dinner and asked me to go to the movies. My mother was out of town, and my father and I had been cleaning up the kitchen when the phone rang. Pleased at the invitation, I told my friend that I could be ready in fifteen minutes and I'd wait out beside the mailbox for her to pick me up. My father, however, grumbled in the background, and so I put my hand over the receiver and asked, "What's up?"

"Well, you haven't asked my permission to go to the movies," my father answered, frowning and raising his voice. "How do I know that your homework is done?"

Turning back to the phone, I told my friend I couldn't go and then hung up, fuming.

"I didn't say you couldn't go," my father said. "I just said you have to ask."

I didn't want to ask, however, and was insulted at his insistence. "I would never agree to go to the movies if my homework weren't done," I said before I flounced out of the room. And this was true. I was god-awful responsible, diligently applying myself to my books almost every afternoon. Besides, the balance of power and responsibility didn't make sense to me. I had to make daily and hourly decisions that determined whether or not I stayed alive. Couldn't I decide on my own whether or not to go to a movie?

My father, I think, simply felt rejected. The very thing that might have made us closer—his participation in my diabetes regimen, which might have brought him understanding of its wider implications for me—hung beyond our reach. On the other hand, I think he hesitated to discipline me as he might have otherwise. This led to a spiraling frustration on both our parts, which never let up until I went away to college.

During those years when I argued with my father at home, I fought with Mr. Houser and Mr. Gilbreath at school. I was the worst kind of troublemaker. By this I don't mean that I did a lot of drugs, or drove the car drunk, or became promiscuous, or skipped classes, or failed to do my homework. In fact, I didn't even smoke cigarettes out behind the gym. I think school officials find those things much easier to deal with than my kind of self-righteous challenges to authority. I didn't respect some of my teachers, and I didn't hesitate to let them know it.

Poor Mr. Houser had been a fundamentalist preacher before he decided to get his teacher's certification for high school math. A thin, rangy, and frankly homely man, he sported long, furry sideburns and polyester leisure suits. The ones in paler colors— one white and one a dull yellow—showed the lines of his underwear and the porcupine chunk of keys in his front left pocket. His speech was peppered with grammatical errors, double negatives, and Appalachian dialect, charming and authentic perhaps in a neighbor or acquaintance, but insulting and comic in school, even a semi-rural public school in Tennessee. His first year of teaching, I had him for sophomore-year geometry.

On the first day of class, from deep sockets under shaggy eyebrows, his black eyes glared with an intense suspicion. Clearly, we were all sinners.

Soon enough, the boys in the class were torturing him accordingly. Spitballs were the weapon of choice, and they flew regularly every time Mr. Houser turned to the chalkboard to demonstrate a proof. "You'uns better stop that," he would say, "or they'll be punishments." For weeks he seemed to expect those retributions to strike us from heaven, turning his face up toward the ceiling tiles with a resigned frown. God, however, did not seem to be on Houser's side, and he grew increasingly agitated.

By this time, everyone was bored and hated geometry. We longed for the days of Algebra I with the wry and tough Mrs. Jones. We whispered and passed notes, and the boys continued tossing spitballs, sometimes adding bits of silly putty or gum to the mix. Mr. Houser decreed total silence in the room and separated me and Jil Fletcher into seats set off from the rest of the class and each other. When the spitballs reached an apotheosis one particularly damp and suffocating winter day, Mr. Houser slammed his fist into his desk and took vengeance into his own hands. For homework we were to copy five hundred words—he suggested from the Bible or the dictionary—and this punishment would remain in force every day that there were spitballs in the air. Those of us innocent of throwing things objected, but to no avail. Girls, we found, would be punished individually for whispering or passing notes or even for our facial expressions, but the boys' behavior meant punishment for all.

The passage I selected for copying originated in a tiny paperback called *The Little Red Schoolbook*, the translation of a handbook for radical students in Sweden. Its thesis was that strict and authoritarian teachers are really just afraid. Mr. Houser, needless to say, was not pleased. He assigned me—and me alone—to copy out a thousand words the night after he returned our "homework."

"You told us it didn't matter what we copied," I objected.

"I can give any student whatever homework I think they need," he smirked.

I copied out another thousand words from *The Little Red Schoolbook*, prepared to give him the entire contents, including the chapters on free sex and drug use. After that, I would mine the Bible for passages on justice, starting with "Vengeance is mine, saith the Lord." Then I thought I might transcribe his lectures in class and provide a commentary on his English usage. I settled in for the long haul.

The next day, however, Mr. Houser called me to the front of the room. I could tell he was going to try to make an example of me, to intimidate me in front of my peers, but I also knew that, as a "smart girl," I would never again be so well loved by my class-mates. The silence in the room was one of anticipation, rather than the usual repression, and I could feel everyone leaning for-ward behind me. Mr. Houser did not stand up, but hid behind the desk. His hands quivered on the papers and his nostrils flared like those of a panicked horse.

"I don't like your attitude . . ." he began.

"My attitude?" I interrupted incredulously. "Well, I don't like yours."

Instantly, his chair bucked to the floor behind him, and he rose, his arm flying through the air as though to smack me in the face. I flinched, but his hand missed my nose and extended toward the door. "In the hall. Now," he ordered. A giggle emanated from Jil in her corner, and he swirled toward her. "You too," he said.

There were all kinds of deliberations about what to do with us. Mr. Houser insisted that he could not allow us to return to his class, but we were both college-bound and our parents insisted that we receive instruction in geometry. Finally, Mrs. Jones agreed to supervise our completion of the course, and Jil and I worked in the library, peacefully, the rest of the year. Mr. Houser taught one more year and then went back to preaching.

Every time there was trouble at school, my parents would be called into a conference with teachers and administrators. My father announced repeatedly that he was tired of going to school, that he wanted the conflicts to stop. Both my parents staunchly defended me in the principal's office, but by the time I was a senior my mother's beginning-of-the-year admonition was, "Your goal for this year is to keep your mouth shut."

At the time, I never associated any of this with my diabetes. That my behavior was tolerated in part because I had a chronic illness never even occurred to me, and I never played that up, never used it in any consciously manipulative way. In fact, it was never mentioned, at least not within my hearing. Perhaps my parents' reactions would have been just the same regardless of my diabetes. Perhaps my rebellions would have been just as intellectual and self-righteous had I been healthy. I don't know for sure, of course, but my sense is that things would have been quite different.

My father might beg to differ, but I seldom defied authority just for the sake of being "different." I may have been born rebellious, but diabetes taught me the stupidity of rebellion for its own sake, defiance for the sake of being merely different from one's parents. For me it wasn't a matter of rebellion against authority for the purpose of being cool with my friends, that standard "us versus them" of adolescence. Rather, I learned early that demands for conformity can be greater from one's peers than from parents—that hippies are no less doctrinaire than yuppies; ravers and punks no less so than Southern Baptists; beer-drinking buddies no less than physicians. I found the tyranny of school cliques as intolerable as that of authority figures.

When my brother graduated from high school, at the end of my junior year, our friend Susan threw a party at her parents' cabin on the lake. Most parents from this crowd thought the party would be supervised, but Susan's parents had discreetly gone out of town, and we would be completely on our own— thirty or forty seventeen- and eighteen-year-olds winding down back roads to the edge of an expanse of black water and brambled woods already thick with the leaves of summer. Waiting for us there were the five-room cabin, a keg of beer, bottles of bourbon and rum, a couple of bags of marijuana, some Quaaludes and speed, a wide lawn down to the water, a rickety dock, several canoes, and one speedboat.

The afternoon before the party, my mother sat down with my brother and me, wearing her serious-talk expression. "I don't want you to try to come home tonight," she said, much to our surprise. "My thinking is that you can get drunk, you can get stoned, you can even get laid, and you can get over it, but if you get killed in a wreck driving under the influence, there is no recovery. So just stay there." My mom, eminently practical, had prioritized the dangers. Still, I arrived home before midnight.

Even then, though my friends might be crazed for this party, might find it the height of high school fun and the ultimate escape from parental dominance, it bored me. Even then, I had no interest in being pawed by drunken boys or in throwing up in the weeds at the edge of the trees. Though I enjoyed getting tipsy, I could not imagine anyone intentionally bringing on a stupor or unconsciousness. I had been that way too many unpleasant times from hypoglycemia to embrace drunkenness. From the position of observer, I watched my friends act stupid.

Susan's brother Michael, beer bottle in hand, led a brigade down to the speedboat, and a chorus of shrieks lifted into the sky over the lower sound of its engine starting. After it lurched away, the waves sloshed the dock, urging to action those kids left on shore, who took up one squirming girl and tossed her into the muddy water. Sputtering and laughing, she dragged herself out and began chasing the others in slow, loopy trails across the grass, like a butterfly moving from one to the next. Finally, in a crescendo of giggles, she collapsed with one boy on top of her wet form, and they wiggled against one another while everyone else drifted back toward the cabin. Inside, the crowd and the smoke thickened as Jimmy Buffett blared from the speakers and doors slammed upstairs. One guy I usually liked dribbled beer down my cheek and slurred a few words into my ear. I knew I was supposed to be thrilled, but I just wasn't.

"Ya like me, don'ya?" he whispered, staggering against me and planting one arm on the wall behind me.

I looked him in his bleary face, put a distancing hand on his shoulder, and said, "Not right now."

I went home, ever divided from normalcy, with no place to fit, neither a goody-two-shoes nor a partying gal.

Needless to say, I gave up on doctors for a while. During college, I never saw one, only the nurse at Student Health in order to obtain a diaphragm or antibiotics for a sinus infection. Oh, perhaps during summer vacation my mother would drag me to Dr. Gilbertson's office for a blood sugar test, but basically I went on about my business without paying much attention to my diabetes. In fact, I more or less quit testing my urine for sugar.

Instead, I developed even further the inward attention that allowed me to "just tell" how I was feeling, a risky business at best. If thirsty and sluggish, I had let my sugar run too high; if shaky or nervous, I knew it was too low. I played it all by how I felt and by being fairly consistent with my habits. I might occasionally eat a few chocolate chip cookies or drink a few beers at a party, but I never skipped injections and I ate regular meals at fairly regular times.

These two habits were probably what staved off blindness and other complications, but they didn't make the quandaries of diabetes any less. At times, I realized, I might be hypoglycemic, I might be completely out of my mind and desperately in need of direction. At others, I needed just as desperately to assert my own sense of things, to say no to doctors, teachers, parents, friends. My rebellion was always tempered by self-questioning, but there were certain points about which I could not afford to conform. Deciding when I could compromise was the hard part, and it became involved in just about every decision I had to make.

My recalcitrance has been a way of saying, all these years, "Why me?" What did I do to deserve diabetes? And if the answer was "nothing," then what other injustices could I refuse in a way I couldn't refuse the illness? Plenty.

When my white friends in Memphis didn't play with black kids, I chose a smiling brown girl named Suzette as my playground favorite.

When the boys at a weekend church retreat tortured and killed a crayfish they'd found in the creek, I wouldn't speak to any of them again.

I may have fought Mr. Houser, but when old Mrs. Blackman, the art teacher, with her halo of frizzy, stark white hair and her wrinkled map of a formerly tanned face, became the subject of tricks, I defended her and made the culprits return the art supplies they'd stolen.

When I found myself, through accident and last-minute changed plans, living with three lesbians my junior year of college, I stayed on principle, even though it made me nervous, even though I faced my own social fallout.

When I caught one of my boyfriends sleeping around, I called all the women in his Rolodex to inform them.

Whenever the boss got unreasonable—changing shift assignments at the last minute in restaurants, demanding too much overtime and asking us to spy on each other's errors at a type-setting shop, taking credit for others' ideas at a design firm, requesting half-truths in ad copy—I quit my job.

When my father left my mother, after twenty-seven years of marriage, I bawled him out.

I picked up litter in the Smoky Mountains, I recycled, I turned off the lights, turned down the heat, worked at the food co-op, ate low on the food chain, donated to charity, tutored people in GED classes, volunteered at the hospital, at the arts council shop, at the animal shelter—all to try to put the wrong world to rights. If something was crazy or cruel, I wanted to stop it. Of course, this made me sometimes crazy or cruel myself, or even funny in a Don Quixote sort of way.

A few years ago, as I strolled down a long, airy mall of elm trees on the campus of the university where I had just taken up residence, I spied a boy—twelve or thirteen years old—tormenting squirrels. It was summer, and the campus was half-deserted, an attitude of bored idleness permeating the humid atmosphere. I was walking home from work, to my suffocating, two-room, phoneless, temporary apartment, and I sweated through my shirt in the heat. Troubled and stressed by the difficult relationship that had brought me to this town and the hassles of a complicated move, I nonetheless felt optimistic that things would get better. I daydreamed about the house we would soon move into, about being together again with my boyfriend and cats, about creating a life in an intellectual community.

The boy appeared like a bad omen, and only gradually did I realize what he was doing, even though the loud bangs had already startled me from my cotton-wool cocoon. He moved in what seemed an erratic arc across a wide expanse of lawn edged with buildings and groups of bushes and trees, toward the mall of

elms under which I walked. I had heard a couple of pops, followed by laughter, and marveled at kids' ability to entertain
themselves, before I saw what he was doing. He would approach
a squirrel, proffering a peanut in one hand, holding a blown-
up balloon in the other. When the squirrel began to gnaw at
the food, the boy, with one determined clap, exploded the balloon right beside the animal, which, of course, ran off terrified.
Cackling, the boy would chase it, stomping at its tail until it got
up a tree.

He was on the fourth squirrel that I'd observed when I
accosted him with such virulence that he must have felt it in his
bones. "What is wrong with you?" I asked as I swooped in like a
hawk. "Picking on harmless, defenseless little animals!"

At first he looked as though he would tell me to bug off, but I
continued, and his shock held him in place, though he looked
over his shoulder once or twice as if calculating whether or not
he could outrun me to the more populated street down the hill. I
delivered an entire little speech on the implications of practicing
cruelty, how it would make him a Nazi or a serial killer. "Do you
want to end up like Ted Bundy or Jeffrey Dahmer?" I threatened
him. "If you don't want to be a criminal, or at least an asshole,
you should get in the practice of being kind."

"Okay, okay," he nodded, swallowing guiltily and hanging his
head ever so slightly. By this time, my anger had dissipated, and
yet he stood patiently, as though waiting for my further instructions, the red balloon now shriveled in his fingers. We eyed each
other, both embarrassed, both caught. And then I told him to get
out of there, which he obligingly did, slinking off down the street
almost as flat to the ground as a railroad track.

I laugh at this story now, for it paints me as a well-meaning
lunatic. While it is crucial to my survival at times, at other times

my toughness goes over the top and twists my intentions as much as any evil would. It also protects a soft, even frightened, core. I had a lot of nerve sassing my father, standing up to my teachers, evoking the ire of my friends and my peers in general, risking becoming an outcast, but there was also in my action a sheer inability to bear the crude posturing of others, the rough and tumble of social interaction, the vicissitudes of life. I developed the habit of challenging other powers, other injustices— especially those I felt affected me—because I was powerless against my disease. I wanted more than anything to be well, to belong, but I knew I never would. Even now, try as I might, I cannot forgive the flawed world. It is no fairer a place than it was the day I got sick.

3

Traveler's Aid

Most of my first trips away from home without parental or grandparental supervision took me into the dense, green wilderness of the Smoky Mountains, along winding trails leading farther and farther into the ever-expanding forest with its secretive ravines and rhododendron thickets. People disappeared in them from time to time—hikers, fugitives, battered women, children once on picnics with their families—and if they were gone longer than an hour or two only rarely were their remains ever found. Someone with a health condition like diabetes would be at a distinct disadvantage in terms of survival if ever lost in this lush indifference, but no one ever balked at my going out into it, only at my going alone.

My brother might spend three nights on a solo excursion as part of his training in the Youth Conservation Corps, but I must always be accompanied on overnights. The few times I ever slipped away on a lone day hike, my small pack laden with bottles of juice and tubes of instant glucose, I would constantly look over my shoulder, unable to shake the sense of someone behind me, watching.

Of course, few people spend much time in the mountains alone, and there are plenty of good nondiabetic reasons for that—broken bones, bears, and rapists are, after all, a danger to anyone. Fortunately there were always passels of teenagers packing up sleeping bags, tiny Coleman stoves, dehydrated beef stew, and contraband cigarettes for a weekend in the Smokies. The mountains were a glorious playground, providing a space in us for a combination of awe at the authority of nature and pleasure in our own growing sense of freedom and mastery. With our parents miles away, we were loosed on the world, sleeping under the stars with the wind riffling through the treetops, naming the constellations as if for the first time, breathing in the openness of the future.

I, however, could become a dependent child again at any moment, and someone always had to be looking out for me. My awareness of this then was dim, as was my association between poor physical function and diabetes. In my family, we simply never blamed anything on the disease. The party line stood firm: you can do anything you want to do, as long as you control the disease rather than letting it control you.

Usually the task of herding me fell to my brother, two years older and a totally responsible kid. In my memory he often plays this managerial role, hovering with a concerned look on his face, eyes reading me to see if I was going under, a slight mistrust in the angle of his inquisitive brow. Because I skipped first grade, having learned to read along with Kelly, one of us on each side of the book my mother held on her lap, we were separated by only one grade in school. Our friends and social lives overlapped considerably—we rode to school together, played cards with a couple of friends every few nights, and did a lot of hiking.

I don't think my presence seemed like too much of a burden. One thing about my family's philosophy about it all was that *no one* dwelt on my condition much. It became part of the overall pattern, woven in with all the other factors of planning a camping trip or other activities. Although my responsibility for myself—and the shame of dependency and hypochondria—had been inculcated in me even before my diabetes, it grew alongside and tangled up with the Christian belief in helping others. Clearly, one wanted to be on the giving (read: superior) rather than the receiving end of assistance, but some give and take was readily acknowledged as proper by my family.

On one trip, I even had to take care of my brother.

Early spring breathes a changeable, fragile air on the Smokies, and backpacking in March and April varies from splendid to snowy. Sunny days, you may sweat and swat gnats from your eyes, but at night when the mists creep through the valleys the chill can be intense. A little overloaded with the winter gear we might need, Kelly and I set out along Big Creek for two nights and three days among the barely fuzzed trees of March. The first day was easy—six miles along the clear, musical stream on the firm, smooth remnants of an old logging road to reach Walnut Bottoms, where the white bark of the walnut trees gleamed in the green surround and we lay, each on our own boulder out in the creek, soaking up the last afternoon light, occasionally sitting up to point out a trout or a water bug or a bird or to plunge a hand or foot into the clear, freezing burble. Ah, peace, rest, sounds worth listening to.

The second day we headed up along a steep, creek-hopping

trail, gaining twice the elevation of the day before in only four miles before reaching the Mount Sterling Ridge Trail at Pretty Hollow Gap. There a carpet of pale hepatica bloomed along a low-slung woodland floor that would soon be too shadowed by tree leaves for such showy displays. We rested before setting out on the last couple of miles along the high, dry ridge to the unused fire tower atop Mount Sterling, our goal and apotheosis.

There is nothing like the sensation of height to allow one to feel godlike, and once there we shed the earthly weight of our packs and clambered up the long flights of stairs to the top of the tower and looked out on the mountains' expanse below. The Smokies, ancient low mountains covered to their tops in thick vegetation, boast few vistas as spectacular as those from Mount Sterling. The mountains stretched out in front of us, huge yet tiny at this distance, indifferent and mysterious, but possessed now by our respectful sight. Kelly and I lingered long, circling our vision from Mount Cammerer, leaning over the Pigeon River gorge to our north and east, across the rolling southern valleys of Cataloochee and around to the imposing peak of Mount Guyot, the sun already beginning to blink from behind its mass in the western sky.

Soon it would be dark, and we hadn't made camp or restored our water supplies yet. We scrambled down and fell to our tasks. Once the tent was up, I gathered sticks and dead limbs for the fire, while Kelly headed off to find the spring that was purported to be just a few hundred feet on down the trail. By the time he came crashing back through the trees in the chilly dark, I was worried and he was irrational, unable to start the camp stove and cursing under his breath as he fumbled around the campsite. I told him to sit, started the stove, and soon put into his cold hands a cup of hot cocoa. Soon enough, the circulation in his fingers and brain was restored, our campfire threw out its zone of warmth, and a pot of noodle soup bubbled on the stove.

"You must've had a low blood sugar," I said, and grinned at Kelly, and he nodded, though both of us were aware that what he'd probably suffered was dehydration.

This became a joke and a shorthand in my family—whenever anyone got weary and depleted to the point of dysfunction, we said that he or she was "having a low blood sugar." This was part of a normalization both true and false, both blessing and curse— a widespread attempt by others to understand, to relate to, but sometimes to dismiss the importance of my illness. The condition of helplessness, temporary and unusual for others, was constant and permanent for me, though certainly less imposing than for my second cousin Cathy, born a spina bifida baby. I grew more and more aware of how health and dependence spread along a spectrum, but remained confused about where I was along that chain. Now I think that diabetes represents the perfect middle: a condition with you forever that will almost certainly limit your life and eventually kill you, but which, if you accept some lifestyle adjustments, allows the appearance of good health and normalcy. It constitutes a tightly balanced catch-22. When I was younger, I only knew that I had to think about diabetes every minute of every day in order to maintain the appearance of not being ill at all.

This generally undramatic character of diabetes—hypoglycemic reactions are relatively rare—and its lifelong duration both contribute to people's mistaken sense that it is no big deal. The greatest compliments to me have always been to the effect that I don't allow my diabetes to interfere with what I want to do; the greatest hurts have come when someone implies or states outright that I've used it as an excuse. These days I long for someone to be impressed with how well I accept the limits. This is a far harder thing to do than struggling against them, but I have *never* heard anyone praise it. People, perhaps rightly, fear the obligations that my weakness implies for them.

The responsibility that fell on my brother especially during those hiking trips, as it would fall on others in other situations later, weighed on him. The speed with which we grew apart after going our different ways to college, I think, reflects his relief at leaving his pseudo-parental role and my resentment of his superiority—physical, academic, and social. Certainly my brother's IQ was higher than mine long before my diabetes, but I nonetheless often wondered what I might accomplish, whether my personality would blossom, if only I didn't have the disease. I didn't want to need help, and I chafed at the very real limitations it put on my life. At the same time, though my brother didn't have the disease, he was stuck with me.

Almost every relationship I've ever had—no matter how slight or how close—has contained an element of the tension first noted with my brother, though it seldom has been articulated as such and it plays out in infinitely various ways. Unlike with more acute illnesses, where the crisis comes and passes, my need is woven into every day that I am also an independent, intelligent, rather stubborn person. The help offered—like the need for it—is various, sporadic, and unpredictable. While most of my childhood friends learned the "rules" and fussed at me if I indulged in anything sweet, Aimee, my zoologist housemate, helped me adjust to the new flexibility in the '80s—she loved to run experiments on my blood sugar with a series of tests before and after a walk, a jog, a donut. One boyfriend became so sensitive to changes in my temperature and muscle tension that he would wake before me when I had a middle-of-the-night low, and the next lover tried to ensure I wouldn't have those lows by applying the regimen to his own life, preparing meals on a precise schedule and asking after the result of every blood glucose test. Most of the time, people try to help and to understand the tricky competition between normalcy and limitation, but it is hard.

Once, when I worried about the dangers of nighttime hypoglycemia because I was thinking of living alone, my friend William said, "Huh. That would be like me saying I don't want to live in an apartment where the bedroom window is high up because I'm short and if the place caught on fire I wouldn't be able to get out as easily as a tall person."

I wanted to ask him, How many times has your house caught on fire? But I let it go. Life is a struggle for everyone, much more so for many than for me. Besides, if I talked about my burden, I would also imply a heavier burden for those around me. I certainly didn't want to remind anyone of that. It only takes one or two rejections of your need to make you afraid of asking, no matter how many helpful people you've also encountered. And many friends have failed me along the way, certainly without intending to do so and often without even realizing they have, simply because they were not in the habit of recognizing other people's needs or because they had so thoroughly absorbed our culture's denial and hatred of anything hinting at dependence.

On one hiking trip, my brother absent, I was shocked to find that it was not my best friend, Lorri, who helped me, but her brother Ralph. Our group of six had driven into the mountains and headed off up the long series of switchbacks to Gregory Bald, a favorite destination just off Cades Cove, where the flame azaleas atop the mountain were rioting red and orange against the greens and blues of the sky and trees. We munched on gorp and sipped from our water bottles as we climbed, and I must have overdone it with the sweets, for, rather than low blood sugar, likely due to the exercise, I began to have the symptoms of elevated blood sugar. I began to stumble, to feel tired and sleepy with a syrupy lethargy dripping through my veins and clotting my mind.

I simply could not keep up with everyone else and had to pause repeatedly to sit and catch my breath along the narrow trail. I felt immobile and stuporous as a queen bee surrounded by active drones swarming the hillside. After assessing my condition with an impatient, accusatory glance, Lorri chased off after some boy she was interested in dating. I didn't see her again until reaching camp. Her older brother, a nihilistic rebel, who had carved a star into the back of his right hand with a pocketknife some years earlier, was the only one with the patience to dawdle with me. He eased me along the trail, stopping when I stopped, taking my sleeping bag to lighten my load, and chatting amiably about the dense shade of the laurel hell through which we walked. He said that he could see I was on some kind of bad trip. And yet the entire case was eventually chalked up to chivalry on his part and female weakness and manipulation on my part. I had been hanging back in order to get him alone with me, everyone teased. It was true that I carried a terrific crush on Ralph after that. But not before.

Although it still was a little humiliating, it was closer to okay if my diabetic crises cast me into the role of helpless *female*. Everyone in my teenage group was comfortable with that. As a *person*, I felt compelled to independence as much as any healthy individual, but if a male could rescue me the situation seemed outwardly almost normal, as though I were simply a weak female, not a sick person. This kind of veiled deflection of the real problem became common in my life, often irritating me but allowing me to sometimes get help and—when none was forthcoming—to avoid brooding about my illness. I myself denied the extra demands of my disease, blaming rejections and disappointments on sexism, politics, bad luck, fatigue—anything but the diabetes, which was so entwined with who I was and which really did at times render me needier than most.

Other categories of partial and mutual dependence, of course, can be just as real as diabetes, and these pose profound questions for individuals and our society. When is it our responsibility to take care of someone? Who should get food stamps or welfare, and how much? How do we distinguish laziness from exhaustion in others or ourselves? How should I gauge my own personal limitations? If I am black and have failed to receive a promotion three times in a row, is the cause racism or my skills? If I have failed in three or more love relationships, should I give up on that and concentrate on my career or charity work or fitness or whatever? When should we struggle, when accept? What risks are stimulating, which are foolish?

I think of the requirement that those graduating from high school in Seattle learn CPR. Because of this, one's chances of surviving a heart attack are considerably higher there than elsewhere in the country. I think of the statistics that show that the lower-middle classes are more likely to donate to food banks than the upper-middle classes. Those who have needed help are more willing to give it, and communities and cultures express a variety of attitudes toward dependence. Mostly, ours denies it, and almost any sort is considered pathological. If this becomes obvious in dicey travel situations with our friends and family members, traveling among strangers brings it even more into focus—if you pass out in the street, is this a place where someone will help you or not?

There is something about being reduced to helplessness in front of strangers and virtual strangers. When they help you, you love them forever. And yet, you are embarrassed by them, too, for they know about you. They've got your number. They've seen you at your worst and have often responded when your loved ones have been absent. It is an odd kind of intimacy, and you owe them something that you will most likely never have the opportunity to repay.

My first experience of this occurred when, at age fifteen, I went on a high school bus trip to Mexico. The trip had gone well—I had had no need for my well-stocked kit of immodium, antibiotics, and blister remedies, and the regularity of tour-provided meals had made it easy for me to fit in with the group. Educationally, the trip combined sentimental tourism and inevitable encounters with widespread poverty. We had climbed the pyramids, shopped for silver bracelets in Taxco, and wandered the streets of Mexico City trailed by beggar children who shamed and frightened us. Along the roads, children younger than we stood in the dusty glare with iguanas for sale, the huge lizards perched eerily on their heads, their free hands beckoning as we passed. Even in the tourist district, prostitutes leaned from balconies to hoot at the boys, and slim, dark men hung around the hotel doors, their eyes on us girls as loud as the whores' voices. As we exited the cathedral, a child running after her ragged mother paused briefly in midstride, lifted her dress, squatted, and peed in a stream of liquid gold, a stunning contrast to the impermeable gilt of the heavenly interior that we had just visited. Dribbling urine down her legs, she darted on toward the woman who had glanced back but never slowed. Together in our little school group, we were learning.

The trouble began on the day before we were to leave Mexico

City for our return to the border. Our bus driver had fallen ill, and the tour company told our teacher that she would have to be responsible for finding a substitute from a stained and ratty list, which was all they would provide. She spent what seemed like hours at a pay phone while we drank sodas in a café, pinching and poking each other in flirtatious teenage boredom and secretly relieved that soon we would be home.

The next morning our new driver showed up with the bus at the hotel door, and we loaded our luggage into the compartment underneath and straggled onto the vehicle. To our surprise, a small woman and a man sat atop a large cooler at the very back of the bus, and we whispered among ourselves as to who they could be. Our teacher's voice rose in protest to the driver, then subsided, and she turned to explain to us that they were other drivers, needed at the border to meet other buses. No one, of course, believed this, but no one wanted to lose our only driver, either. We sank into our high-backed seats in that state of public transport relaxation: someone else is driving, you are not at the wheel, you might as well enjoy the passing view.

By afternoon, our teacher realized we were not on the right road. Our designated rest stops had never appeared on the signs, our lunch had not materialized, our driver had waved away her questions without answers. Finally, she insisted he pull over, and at a broken-down roadside stand a confrontation ensued, teacher and driver yelling and flailing all over the parking lot, the rest of us sealed inside the bus with the trembling pair in the back. Our driver, it turned out, had never been to the border before, though he had for years driven a city bus. In bad times, he had been laid off and was now hoping to ride this bus all the way into the United States with his wife and brother—sitting in the back on a case of Coca-Cola they hoped to sell on the streets of Laredo to support themselves until they could get other work as illegal aliens. We were, it turned out, on the old road to the border instead of the recently built highway that offered a more direct route.

"It's all right," the teacher said with an uncertain sigh. "This will get us there. It will just take a little longer. When I was in college we used to go this way." She had not told the driver that Mexican buses stopped at the border, that we would board a different one there, with an American driver, before crossing. Assured that she would not turn him in to the law, the Mexican driver pulled the bus back out onto the road and headed north.

I ate the last of my store of packaged peanut butter crackers for lunch, knowing that it was the last food on the bus. We had all planned to stock up at our rest stop, with its American-like store of convenience foods and its soothing lack of lurking men. There had been no open stores along this route, this cracked and abandoned trail through the desert. I knew I would be in trouble soon, but I stayed put, the sun glowering through the windows to my left, the voices of my friends raised in camp-song frenzy, the hands on my watch sweeping round and round.

Some hours later, as darkness fell and in the middle of a verse of "Grandma's Feather Bed," I called to the teacher to tell her that I was slipping into insulin shock. In those days, I took a type of insulin that you injected once a day—its suspension was designed for three peaks of action, one for each of three very regular and traditional meals. That insulin was in me, waiting to act, before we'd even left Mexico City. Now, with it nearing 9 P.M., I was way past due for the carbohydrates that insulin was intended for, pale and shaking, with my neck wavering like a weak stem. The teacher surveyed the other students to make sure no one secreted any snacks, and then, swiftly, her eyes sure as a missile-tracking device, she turned to the back of the bus, to the case of Cokes underneath our special guests.

With a stream of Spanish as urgent as a siren and her hands flapping like a flag in a gale, she babbled to them. She was poised for ferocity, and, idly, I thought about her own raging hysterical personality, how she loved telling the story of how a Mexican had tried to rape her but she had poked one of his eyes out, how we ourselves cowered in front of the knobby attenuation of her pointing fingers. I was afraid she would garble things, but her "Without one, she may die" was clear enough. Immediately, both of the pair stood and bent to lift the lid, handing her not one, but two of the bottles from their store.

Without a word, the teacher came back toward the front of the bus, handed me the drinks, and passed on back to her seat as though she had gone to the bathroom and her business was done. She didn't ask me if I was all right until after we had changed buses at the border, leaving our Mexican acquaintances behind, and were unloading in the parking lot of Denny's, where we would eat our first meal in more than fourteen hours.

But those people had given me a Coke, those people with nothing in the world but hope and a case of sodas to sell on the sidewalk. I wished that I could have given them a home, a few dollars, at least my thanks, but my teacher forbade me to speak to them. The woman had smiled at me when I looked back toward her, the bottles in my hands, and had flipped her hand upward, gesturing, "Go ahead. Drink." We were fellow travelers in an unpredictable universe—she too knew that. For a long time I imagined them stranded in Nuevo Laredo, trying to get back to Mexico City through the wide desert with their cooler, or dying of dehydration after slipping under the fence into the United States, their act of kindness to me dissolved into the starry sky.

· · ·

At age thirty-six, I finally went to France, barely escaping the fate of Lucy Jordan, a haunting character in a Marianne Faithfull song, who went mad when she realized that her dull fate would forever exclude driving around Paris. At last, at long last, I entered the City of Love, of wine and fine cuisine, of Notre Dame and the Louvre, of Cézanne, the American expatriate writers, Foucault and Kristeva, of citizens with aesthetic and intellectual soul—the center of all kinds of things that were central to me. Everyone I knew had told me over and over, for years and years, that I would love Paris, and I did. Why had it taken me so long to get there?

My father, I think, disliked travel and thought it basically frivolous. In the early years, we went on vacations, mostly camping and to our relatives' homes, once to Florida and Disney World, once to Myrtle Beach, once on a big trip to Philadelphia and Washington, often to historical sites around the South— Brices Cross Roads, Chickamauga, Natchez Trace. I saw the West Coast for the first time during high school, on a trip to visit colleges my brother might attend, combined with a professional conference of my father's in Montana and a stopover at a family friend's in Colorado. For both my parents, professional activities, education, and keeping up relationships with family and friends certainly all took precedence over travel for its own sake. Amazingly, my parents paid cash for two very expensive, private-college educations for my brother and me, and this was definitely more important than ski trips to Vermont, or renting condos at the beach, or even going to the Grand Ole Opry. (We didn't get cars for high school graduation, either.) My mother never traveled outside the United States before their divorce, and my father, though his own mother was an inveterate taker of tours and went all over Europe, to the Middle East, India, and Japan, has still been no further than Alaska. That, too, was a working trip.

Later, spending a weekend at Whistler Mountain ski resort with a boyfriend and his college buddies, appalled at the expense and decadence of the village full of pricey shops and the bars full of drunken and obnoxious revelers, I wondered if my family had just been too serious. I looked around at the waste of the place, at how the mountain had been shorn and blasted and strung with wires, cables, and harsh buzzing lights, how the wildlife had been driven off in order to create a playground for adults, and I was offended. The long rides to the top, the parades of gear and fancy skiwear, the repetitive swoops to the bottom again, the games of Quarters in the bar, beer splashing everywhere and conversation a dull roar of idiocies, all seemed worse than useless to me. But everyone else seemed to be having a great time, and it occurred to me that I'd just never learned to have fun.

Within a complex matrix of reasons, a certain carefree attitude has always evaded me, and I have felt like an impostor when I was doing anything but working in some form or another. Most of my friends in high school and college, though certainly not all, separated their work and pleasure in ways foreign to me. They drank more, they drove faster, they dated people they didn't even particularly like, they undertook hobbies such as Dungeons and Dragons, tennis, the Society for Creative Anachronism, hang-gliding, collecting rubber stamps, shopping at flea markets, crashing through the woods on mountain bikes or motorcycles. They loaded up in cars and drove to Florida for spring break. They hitchhiked around Germany and lived with families in Pau and photographed mating turtles in the Galapagos and danced with one-armed men in Jamaica and stumbled ill through the streets of Cairo and trailed their fingers in the blue, blue water from catamarans off the shore of Cypress. Even my brother married into a family that owns and spends frequent weekends at a ski condo in Vermont and a beach house on Cape Cod.

Alternately, I have envied and despised such privileged postures, as does anyone who watches a parade of the unattainable but questions the value of the prize: the teenager who murders for Nikes that may be the wrong size, the woman who starves herself trying to be as thin as Cindy Crawford, the black man who can't shake his obsession with blondes.

Discouraged from traveling—or even from being—alone, I nonetheless could not travel—or go—along with whatever happened because a running picture of dangerous possibilities played in my head. I can't help but think that my sensitivity to consequences, a major component of my serious nature, came at least in part from my disease. My vigilance could never end. And my constant duty involved a fortune-telling worthy of a psychic: If I eat this, what will happen in an hour, in two? If I don't eat it, will I pass out? What time will my friends want to stop for lunch? If we take off on foot, how many calories will I expend? Will everyone want to walk all afternoon, or will they grow tired and want to take a bus home? Will the temperature outside drop, increasing my need for carbohydrates? How much food and juice do I need to carry with me? What happens if the car breaks down or if the airplane is delayed on the runway? I had to be prepared for every contingency, as my health literally depended on it.

I learned this fear for my life through osmosis, I think, as we never talked about it in my family as such. But in Paris it came home to me that such fear must have pervaded my growing up.

I went to France with my mother, almost a year after the sudden death of her second husband. She had proposed the trip as something for her to look forward to between his death in June and the following May when we would go, as a break in her difficult professional life and as a reward for all my hard work in graduate school. Not long after my parents' divorce, she and a gentleman friend of hers had gone to Paris, and it had been revelatory enough for her that now she considered it a gap in my own education that I had not seen Europe. Avidly, with endless enthusiasm, with a determination to see as much as possible in our two short weeks, and with a longing and sense of lack I'd never before realized I had, I pored over the books, garnered advice from all the travelers I knew, and planned itineraries for the Champs-Elysées and the Louvre, the Left Bank and Latin Quarter, Père Lachaise Cemetery, the Place Vendôme, the Musée d'Orsay, the Eiffel Tower, Montmartre, the Pompidou Center, Versailles, Chartres, Chenonceau in the Loire Valley, and Giverny. I wanted to make up for lost years.

But there is no way to make up for lost years, at least not completely. Let's face it: I was thirty-six years old and with my mother on a baldly tourist agenda. I was not going to experience the Paris nightlife or have even mild flirtations after sitting in cafés reading Gide or Rilke or Proust. I would not be invited to any artists' ateliers or gallery openings, nor would my French become fluent. Not as ostentatious as typical Americans, my mother and I would be continually taken for English. I felt dowdy and doughy, sleepy-faced and with feet as wide as the Seine. I had a hard time shaking off the romantic movies and enjoying the Paris I was actually in.

All the old tensions about burden and responsibility—denied and reduced and beaten into a buried cell by my years of living by myself—returned with as much cacophony as if the ghosts of Marie Antoinette and Gertrude Stein had tried to dance

together. Used to living with at least the appearance of independence, I churned in the face of my mother's ministrations.

Outside Père Lachaise, near the Métro stop on Boulevard de
Ménilmontant, in a cold, gray wind and a surging flux of com-
muters, we reached a crisis. A couple of days earlier, we'd had a
wonderful afternoon perusing the cemetery, both enchanted with
the vast hillside of tombs crowded together in their final sociability, the famous and the obscure elbow to elbow under the ground
and the elaborate marble; paths meandering among the hedges,
trees, statues, and monuments as gently as through any village.
From Heloise and Abelard to Jim Morrison, the dead greeted us
in their quiet ways. We had wandered among the various pasts of
Paris for several hours, until the daylight faded.

I wanted to go back for several reasons. First, I had run out of
film without a photo of Proust's grave, and, perhaps childishly, I
wanted such a token of proof and solidarity with this invalid
writer from whom I had learned so many lessons of style and
insight. Then, too, I hoped that to visit a place a second time
would create a sense of familiarity that, as a casual tourist and
rank amateur, I might not otherwise experience, a second sight
that would allow me to see a little deeper. Also I simply felt like
walking alone for a while, not matching my mother's pace, not
looking over my shoulder, but moving like a shark's fin through
water or a hound on a scent—according to an internal focus,
swift, erratic, undeterred.

Since we had already scoped out the Père Lachaise neighborhood and the subway route, it seemed to me as though this made
perfect sense as a time when my mother might stay at the hotel
or a coffee shop and rest out of the chilly spring wind, writing postcards or reading up on what she might want to do that
afternoon. We had been going at quite a pace, after all, and

her stamina had been lowered by a difficult year at work and all the emotional and practical traumas following the death of her husband.

The Wednesday morning I'd picked to retrace to the cemetery blew up particularly raw and drizzly, and over café au lait and croissants at the hotel I suggested that my mom stay in while I venture out. Nothing doing. She said she'd at least accompany me to the neighborhood and that then we could go directly to Montmartre for the afternoon. So we clambered onto a Métro car and headed off, me recalling the pleasant café with its warm red awnings at the bottom of the hill near the cemetery gate, she planning to stick as close to me as pantyhose. As soon as we stepped into the wind from the Métro exit, our cross-purposes came clear.

"It's a huge place," my mother said, her face contorted with concern and the tip of her nose reddening in the cold, "and empty. You don't know what kind of . . . elements there are in there. You don't know the language. This is a foreign country. What if someone wants to rob you? What if you get lost? What if you have . . . a low blood sugar?"

I tapped the purse strapped across my torso. "There's more instant glucose in here than money," I smiled firmly. "Besides, you have to understand, most of my friends came to Europe all by themselves when they were twenty. I'm thirty-six, and you don't want me to cross the street by myself. I can't stand that."

My mother began to gulp and sniffle, the tears streaming sideways from her eyes, parallel to the wind-whipped fringes of her scarf. At the time I didn't even think about how she might be afraid for herself alone in an alien city, how her sense of loneliness and vulnerability might be heightened by Owen's death, or how she might want me to take care of her. I just assumed she was being overprotective of me.

From the beginning of the trip, we had rocked back and forth in an uneasy, shifting balance of strengths and weaknesses—my mother had the authority of money, age, and parenthood; I had the energy of a younger person and a slight edge on the language and practical details. In truth, however, our conflicts had gone beyond these issues, and we had found ourselves grappling with larger changes in our relationship: her diminished state transferred more of the burden of care to me, and for us this was definitely new. My mother had always seemed invincible. She had trained me to be independent of everyone but her.

By this I don't mean to imply some sort of pathological domineering parenting, not at all, for my mother had sent me out into the world, had respected my stubborn desires, and had remained my staunchest supporter in spite of all my mistakes and disagreements with her. In many ways, I was independent of her too, but I had been a chronically ill child, and my mother had continued always to carry the responsibility of being there if and when I needed help. No one questions this during childhood, and I have long wondered why people expect this closeness to disappear as soon as an ill or disabled child turns eighteen. In Paris, it frightened me to see that she might weaken, that she might not always be there, and that, in fact, I might need to face the usual shift that takes place when one's parents age.

In a knot of irritation, I feared both growing up and not growing up, and she feared both still being responsible for me and growing old. I remembered my mother's words after her own father's death: "There's grief, and that's one thing," she said, "but there's also knowing that you are on the front lines. The next turn will be yours." I had always, somewhat reasonably, expected my mother to outlive me. *Steel Magnolias* was the only public example I had.

We stood on the street in Paris, ashamed and frustrated. Still angry, but determined to put a brave face on things, my mother swallowed the lump in her throat, I patted her arm and reassured her that it would be fine, we agreed on a time I'd be back, and she headed into the coffee shop while I zipped off up the hillside under the trees, thinking of the passage in Proust, given me as a model by a writing teacher:

> If my health had grown stronger and my parents allowed me, if not actually to go down to stay at Balbec, at least to take, just once, in order to become acquainted with the architecture and landscapes of Normandy or Brittany, that 1.22 train into which I had so often clambered in imagination, I should have wished to stop, for preference, at the most beautiful of its towns . . .

The "ifs," the "just once," and the process of imagining experiences one never will have throbbed with my increased pulse as I climbed—in actuality not fantasy—up the steep path to Proust's austere black slab, an expanse of marble so plain that its main decorations are the reflected images of the overhanging trees and the flowers strewn by admirers over its impenetrable and isolated surface.

There are, I thought, different ways to enrich oneself, and we adapt as best we can to our circumstances. Mirrored experience is one type of reality. Still, there is a wonderful lightness in walking the actual path sometimes, even sometimes alone.

Last September, however, I was not prepared to be abandoned in Italy. At the foot of the burly Dolomites in a tiny village called Castello di Aviano, I found myself unexpectedly alone in a country where my knowledge of the language was limited to the Berlitz guide for travelers, which I had owned for a mere three weeks. In the modest house loaned by an acquaintance, I got up, looped my Medic-Alert charm around my neck, made several panic-stricken and tear-filled telephone calls, walked into the larger town of Aviano, rented a stalwart Opel for two days, and, in order to regain my lost composure, drove up into the mountains with a map and a bag of smelly cheese, stale rolls, and hard fruit candies.

My traveling companion—once a college roommate and a friend for eighteen years—had wanted to ride motorbikes into the Dolomites, over to some wine country near the Slovenian border, perhaps as far as Trieste. I refused. Earlier, we had talked about doing these excursions by car, but that would not do for Sheri now. She and Chris, she said, always got around on motorcycles when they were in Bermuda or Costa Rica. Besides, we had already ridden mopeds around the island of Elba—what was the big deal now?

Rain, I said. On Elba we were always within a few miles of our hotel. And cold. We didn't know what the temperature might do in the mountains in late September. And traffic—I didn't want us to drive into a city like Udine or Trieste with no one to navigate, on two bikes that might be separated with one wrong turn. Besides, Elba represented my first time on a two-wheeled vehicle, and, though I had survived the twisty coastal roads there, I had nearly gone over the cliffs twice. If that happened up in the Dolomites, I pointed out to Sheri, the terrain and language were so unfamiliar that she might not even be able to tell anyone where my unconscious body lay, or that they would need to consider diabetes in any treatment. Who knows what the medical care is like in this part of the world, I said, or where the nearest hospital might be? The risks just seemed too high, when we could do the same thing by car, easily, comfortably, cheaply.

But Sheri would only feel free on a motorcycle. I was holding her back, preventing her from doing as she pleased on her own vacation.

We had been at odds since the beginning of our trip, the spur-of-the-moment five-week train adventure Sheri had proposed to me only a couple of weeks before we departed. Down about a troubled love relationship, I was ripe for escape, and Sheri, a lawyer recently made wealthy by a large case, had offered to pay air and train fare and the bulk of hotel costs. It seemed like a fabulous opportunity for a little-traveled graduate student on a strict budget like me, but Sheri had belittled my paltry Italian, fought with shopkeepers and hoteliers, refused to go to museums, and bragged continually about how being rich would allow her to do anything she wanted. She had little tolerance for my suggestions or needs, and her face had flattened into a mask of continual irritation. For a while, I blamed myself and the requirements of my illness.

Travel is never easy with diabetes. Changes in time zone, unknown ingredients in food served in restaurants, and fluctuating levels of activity can all wreak havoc with the tight balance of blood sugar control. Already, in Paris, waiting for Sheri to arrive before we set out, I had gone into a middle-of-the-night insulin shock so severe that my boyfriend had to revive me by pouring juice down my throat. It was sheer luck that he had decided to pause with me there during his own European jaunt; otherwise I would have awaited Sheri alone and might have been seriously ill before her arrival.

So, when she left me in Aviano, frankly I was scared. To her, the trip together "just hadn't worked out"; in my mind, there was a bit more involved. Still, I had given her permission to leave me there. If there was one thing worse than being alone, risking my health, it was being a drag, restricting someone else's carefree sojourn.

Before I could resume the bustle of train travel and tourist sites, however, I needed to reassure myself, and I turned to the Dolomites to do so. Driving into mountains and finding a winding trail along a lake or stream was something I knew how to do, no matter what the language, and I knew it would restore me. I wound up the narrowing ribbon of pavement away from the hectic valley, turned off into a parking lot with wooden signs, and followed my feet along a misty path toward a glittering, chill body of water. My breath came deep in the silent woods, and I reached that mysterious mixture of alienation and comfort that makes travel fun. Then I was able to lie in the long, blond grass alongside the nameless blue-green lake, the oblique and familiar early autumn sun soothing on my eyelids, the wind clicking in the strange, husky vegetation, my mind happily stirred toward watery Venice and the rest of unknown Italy.

When Sheri and I parted company in Italy, I was certainly glad that I'd spent a couple of hours alone in Père Lachaise the previous year. Of course, Sheri and I hadn't been so continually joined as my mother and I had been—we had agreed to go our separate ways a number of different afternoons, such as when I wanted to visit the Uffizi in Florence and she preferred more time in the shops and cafés. Once I had gathered my wits in Aviano, I was eager to go on by myself, Sheri's fits of pique and paranoia fading like the high whine and gasoline odor of a passing motorbike. I changed the film in my camera from black and white to color, revved up my credit cards, and launched into my new adventure.

My mother had offered to buy me a ticket home right away, but that idea was anathema to me. On one level, my fears seemed ludicrous anyway, as I'd lived alone for the past six years. That most dangerous of diabetic times—the wee hours of the night when one is asleep and least likely to notice the signs of hypoglycemia—would be no different in hotel rooms in Italy than in my bedroom at home. Sure, sure, the disruptions in routine, the difficulty of communication, and my own distraction under the influence of centuries of art and architecture might increase my risks, but, I reasoned, they do that for everyone who travels—who might not encounter a pickpocket or a step to trip over or a bit of tainted food or drink? I was utterly free—how could I not revel in that?

I rode the jam-packed train into Venice in high spirits and had a fabulous first day there—finding my cozy hotel just around the corner from the station, donating my now sapped paperbacks to the desk clerk's collection and chatting with him about books, taking a boat ride with three young men who easily could have robbed me blind and dumped me in the ocean but who instead blushed and smiled and waved when they let me off at the Chiesa della Madonna dell'Orto to see the Tintorettos there, and eating my dinner in a tiny, cheap pizzeria with a group of high school students from Puglia. In a riotous amalgam of their schoolbook English and my Berlitz Italian, we traded information about our itineraries and our lives, and the girls were thrilled to meet "an independent American woman." I laughed and told them that I was afraid of traveling alone, but what could I do? We all laughed, and they told me about the dreams that they were afraid of never achieving.

"I want to be a doctor," one told me, "but my mother wants me to get married and have grandchildren." The boys at the next table hooted halfheartedly, and she shook her head, her short dark curls recoiling, her spine stiff, her face turned away from them.

"*La vita è un* ... river, river—" I philosophized, thumbing through my dictionary. "*La vita è un fiume.* It takes you strange places—*a les postos stranos.*" As I returned to my hotel and went to sleep, I was accompanied by the image of the circle of nodding heads and the memory of our indulgent laughter.

The next evening, near disaster cut through the pleasant hours I'd passed trundling the streets, shops, churches, and museums of Venice. All the way down to San Marco at the tip of the island from my hotel near the train station before sunrise, I had now been on my feet for better than twelve hours, with only the occasional respite of mineral water or coffee in a café. Exhausted, but emboldened by the previous night's success, I stopped early for dinner in a tourist joint with an outdoor patio and agreed readily when two Australian women asked me to join them. But then I made that series of simple errors in judgment that can so easily lead to diabetic trouble.

I had tested my blood sugar an hour or so earlier, and as it had been a comfortable 189 I assumed I didn't need to test again at the dinner table with strangers. An injection would cause enough of a stir. The Australians had already ordered when I sat down, and so, again in order to minimize disruption, I simply asked for the same, and three problems stemmed from the meal. First, it came with wine, which like a fool I drank—considering my own already exhausted state and the unpredictable effect of alcohol on blood sugar wherein it may evoke a precipitous drop. Also, we were early for an Italian dinner—many restaurants don't even open until after seven—and the kitchen was slow in bringing the meal. Since a diabetic needs to take insulin fifteen minutes to a half hour before eating, in order that the peaks of its action and that of food digestion will match, I had taken my shot shortly after the wine was served. The food itself—graciously plentiful in all the other Italian restaurants I'd been in—turned out to be thin and stingy. Even the basket of bread sat out of reach on the other side of the table, and our conversation was animated enough that I didn't interrupt to ask for it.

By the time we left the restaurant, my senses had fuzzed and blurred, and I only dimly knew what went on around me. Twelve hours of constant walking, the alcohol, the delayed and meager meal, and the fact that my mind was crammed with views of water and islands from the campanile; the glittering array of stone and mosaic in San Marcos; Tintoretto, Titian, Tiepolo, and the lovely pastel portraits of Rosalba Carriera; the tombs in the section especially for bambini at San Michele, and the cassocked priest that showed the way to the grave of Ezra Pound—these normal events of travel conspired to render me irrational and nearly unconscious.

My pride also got in the way. I didn't want to admit to my two companions that anything was wrong, though the fact kept trying to claw its way into my consciousness and though, when I had pulled out my syringe, one had exclaimed that her brother also has diabetes. If anyone would have been helpful and understanding, they would have been. Perhaps even more, I didn't want to admit to myself that something was wrong. After all, I had only the day before begun to enjoy the solitary journey, to feel competent again, and here I was crashing, demonstrating my own pathetic inability to take care of myself, my easy vulnerability. As we left the restaurant, I stumbled on the uneven paving stones, and one of the Australian women asked if I was okay. Somehow, I felt ashamed and I wanted more than anything just to get away from them. I told her I was tired and was headed directly back to my hotel. Firmly, I told them good-bye, and soon the bustling crowds of the Strada Nova separated us.

As soon as they were gone, a desperate terror crept over me like a chill from the darkening water all around me, but a terror I could only see far off. It was as though I watched a murder across miles of field, through a pair of malfunctioning binoculars. Was it really a murder or just a fight? Maybe the woman only danced in front of the man, twirling her skirt in joy not flight? Was that really a knife in his hand, or a wineglass shining in the moonlight? Perhaps he only spilled some Chianti down the front of her dress; perhaps she lay on top of him in a lover's huddle and he had not run off leaving her there in the grass. What did I see? What did I feel in my own body? Icy fear for which I hated myself. Confusion which I could not sort out. I wasn't sure in which direction I walked. I couldn't read the signs painted on the walls to keep tourists from getting lost in the Venetian maze. People milled around me, trying to ignore my faltering step.

Finally, my instincts and my long years of diabetic training kicked in: if you know something is wrong, even if—especially if—you can't tell what, you eat something sweet. Automatically. No questions asked. Right now. Still stumbling along, bumping into other people like a rubber ball thrown onstage with a bunch of precise, purposeful dancers, I fumbled through my purse for the glucose tablets I always carried and ate several in quick succession. These increased my awareness enough to make me more afraid, but not much more coherent.

Now all I wanted was to eat everything in sight, but my poor Italian, further wrecked by my hypoglycemia, rendered me terribly offensive to the woman at the gelato stand, which suddenly, as if by Divine Providence, appeared in front of me. In spite of the fact that I had learned and practiced the explanation, "*Ho il diabete, e il mio zucchero dello sangue è basso,*" the words would not come. I could hardly speak. The woman scowled, grabbed the money that I mindlessly proffered, unable as I was to comprehend or count it, and waved her scoop through the air. "*Quale gusto? Quale gusto?*" she demanded. Shrugging and pointing, I persevered enough to get some kind of ice cream cone, which I gobbled down, wondering what the Australian women would think if they happened upon me again.

If they saw that I was in insulin shock, they would wonder why I had not asked for help, why I was being so weird. They might suspect that I'd intentionally taken too much insulin as an excuse to overindulge, or that I was simply "cheating" on my diet, that I had given them the slip in order to overeat without listening to any admonitions about how "you're not supposed to eat *that!*" Pig! Drunk! Secret eater! American idiot! Stupid woman! All around me, people seemed to disapprove, their elbows jostling me, their impersonal faces turning away like flowers from the dark.

As I staggered on, now sweating and feeling sick to my stomach, I began to have intermittent moments of lucidity, at least about my condition. The classic symptoms of low blood sugar that had deserted me on the way down now visited me on the way back up, and I started to shake and to feel freezing cold all the way to the bone. But I couldn't figure out why I wasn't rebounding more quickly—I had eaten, not only dinner but supposedly fast-acting glucose tablets and ice cream. Usually, recovery from hypoglycemia is swift and simple, and so I wondered if something else was wrong, but, but ... I only wondered a moment at a time. My brain was like a light with a three-year-old at the switch—flickering on and off.

Try as I might, I could not concentrate long enough to recognize where I was. Intermittently, I would see—the rim of a gondolier's hat silhouetted against the sunset lingering on a wall, the hand of a mother clasping her kid's arm as they rushed past, a row of glass-bead necklaces hanging behind a window—and then a gray fog would creep across my vision. I'd shake my head, wipe my hand across my face as if to pull the curtain away, blink and blink, but I couldn't see. Then a spot would clear, as though someone were wiping mud off my windshield, and I could see out again for a while.

Enough awareness had returned that I trembled from fear as well as the low glucose. When I found myself teetering precariously near the edge of the Grand Canal in front of the train station, I knew I was close to my hotel, but I still could not find it.

I threw myself at the yellow-and-white vaporetto kiosk, at the uniformed man behind the counter and the Plexiglas shield. "*Aiuto mi,*" I whispered, crumpling forward onto the counter. In a hopeless exercise, my mouth opened and closed, pantomiming speech, but nothing else would come out. On the other side of the glass, the man stood back, his fleshy face swelling in indignation and disgust, his wide fingers spread motionless on the edge of the counter.

People were strolling up behind me to buy tickets, and his eyes flashed angrily between them and me.

I looked over at him, my own fingers clutching at the edge on my side, my knees feeling soggy under the weight of my body, my face flushing in humiliation, my mind a scramble out of which I could form no words.

"*Che cosa desidera? Che? Che?*" I watched his thin lips spit out the words, but I could not understand. His cheeks expanded, then he expelled the air in a heavy sigh through his pursed mouth. Stolid as he stood, his face contorted in a million directions at once. "*Vada via.* Go away," he said.

I flattened my palms on the smooth plastic and finally choked out the name of the hotel. "*Dolomiti,*" I said.

"*Eccola!*" His arm swung into a sudden, harsh, dismissive gesture, toward a point somewhere behind me. His head wagged in disbelief at my stupidity, for right behind me, just a few yards away across the pavement, was a large sign with a prominent arrow pointing the way to my hotel. I was less than a block away.

Seldom have I been so glad to arrive anywhere as I was to achieve my room at the fine little Hotel Dolomiti, where I went through the motions of self-preservation: Stop for the key. Fortunately, the clerk knows your room number, so you don't have to say a word. Climb the six flights of stairs. Manage to get the door open. Drop your purse. Eat a half package of Hit cookies. Collapse into the narrow bed under the swirled Venetian light fixtures. Sleep fitfully with the light on all night, rising from time to time to test your blood sugar again. Look in the mirror to make sure you are really there.

In the morning I felt okay, and the Venetians once again were lovely and kind. Chagrined, I promised myself that I'd have no more alcohol on this trip.

In Ravenna, standing at the bar of the Ca da Ven with the friendly locals offering to buy me drinks, I chose *la acqua minerale*, much to their amusement. In San Giovanni, at the home of the brother and sister-in-law of a friend from home, I accepted one glass of wine with a full dinner, but only because they understood and would be there all night. In Rome, I met two American guys who work and live in Kazakhstan, and one took me to dinner, but I declined to drink the wine, especially since the day felt so much like the fateful one in Venice—I'd toured all day on foot, covering miles of territory in the hot weather, a cool night had fallen, and I was excited and stimulated by congenial conversation in my own language for a change. This time, I would take no risks and the evening would pass with me fully conscious, an odd kind of triumph, but a triumph nonetheless.

I had realized that my whole strategy had to change, that I had to be more serious than usual about the proscriptions attached to diabetes. Mostly, this was just a matter of paying closer attention, thinking about it more, keeping the level of my awareness high. I tested my blood sugar more often, even setting my alarm for 3 A.M. to avoid middle-of-the-night lows, and let it run a little higher than usual—not a good idea for the long term, but for another few days in Italy, a sensible compromise. When I walked, I snacked. And I told almost everyone I met about my diabetes, so that the words would be more familiar to my tongue.

This led to some of the best conversations I had in Italy, for there is nothing that crosses national boundaries like sharing a disease. One waiter in Rome said, "Mi anche, me also," and proceeded to explain to the chef why he must prepare my meal right away in spite of the busy lunch hour. With a flourish and a nod, he set my roast chicken and fava beans before me almost instantly.

On the packed train from Bologna to Chiusi, where I had to transfer to get to San Giovanni, I sat with an older couple—a skinny man with thinning, oily hair and thick, tinted eyeglasses and a large woman in a tight, navy blue polyester dress, her white hair puffed and coiffed with a heavy barrette across the back. They sat across from each other in the window seats, in a conspiracy of bad teeth and dismay that this strange American might invade the space they had staunchly defended so far. The man laid his hand on top of the small bag in the seat beside him, as if to say, "I will not move it. This seat is taken," so I heaved my backpack into the overhead rack and squeezed in beside her.

It was the most crowded and least friendly train I'd been on, and this only seat I could find was smack in the middle of a smoking car full of dingy couples and single mothers screaming *"Basta!"* at their hordes of cramped, bored children smacking and kicking each other across the aisle. It also happened to be lunchtime, and I had carried along a bedraggled focaccia sandwich and a rather bruised apple. Already, as a single, blond American female in a very Italian car, I was the subject of raised eyebrows and turned necks. I could see that I would have a full audience for the performance of my testing and injecting. Inwardly, I sighed and calmed the butterflies in my stomach, hoping that my sincere smile would make everyone more receptive to my poor explanations.

I pulled from my enormous purse the small turquoise-pink-and-purple Peruvian bag that I use to carry meter, test strips, insulin, and syringes, and set it on the fold-out table in front of me. After wiping my hands down my thighs, I unzipped the pouch. All around, people simultaneously ignored and watched to see what I could possibly be doing with that odd little bag. One step at a time, I thought, pulling the plastic meter case out. The man in the seat across from me stared, and so I began my halting explanation, leaning toward him to create the illusion of a conversation.

To my surprise, he and his wife both nodded emphatically as I began the process of getting out a test strip, lancing my fingertip, and lining up the drop of blood. While the machine began its countdown, beeping loudly in the quieted car, the man began to fumble with the squat brown vinyl bag beside him. Then he pulled out his own meter, precisely the same model as mine. We laughed, suddenly allies in this space full of normals.

Throughout lunch, I chatted as best I could with the diabetic man and his wife, who spoke no English, but who were very patient as I paused to look words up in my dictionary, a new addition to the Berlitz guide. In Europe, a different set of measures is used for blood sugar, so we had to negotiate what was "normal" by each standard in order to compare ours. It was easier to go through all the usual stuff—as predictable as the hometown question at college freshman parties—duration of the disease, age at diagnosis, what type of treatment, how often one indulges in sweets. A Type 2 diabetic, he'd only been diagnosed for six years and was still managing with pills and diet, though he might have the occasional cookie. I admitted my weakness for ice cream, and he fussed at me about that while I admonished him for smoking cigarettes. He and his wife were glad that I was on my way to friends in San Giovanni, though they never once questioned my traveling alone.

The entire mob on the train whispered back and forth about what was going on, one woman explaining to another that we were talking about our eating habits, but no one really catching on. We had created quite a stir, and what was lovely was that it didn't even matter. I could be happy to meet these people and to find we had something in common, but the need I felt for their help was social, not medical. I was taking care of myself at last. And I was doing an okay job of it.

"*Buona fortuna, buona fortuna,*" the couple called as I departed the train. "*Arrivederci!*"

Four months after I got home, Sheri called. I wasn't home, but she left a message saying that we'd been friends too long for this disruption to end it. I know she is right. And yet for me there is another meaning in Italy, a meaning beyond our wanting to do different things on our trip. I hesitated to call her back. In order to do so, I have to give up any expectation of care, I have to take complete responsibility for something I cannot always handle. I need to fit myself to normal standards, to set aside my own pressing needs, to keep to myself. It is the inevitable quandary of the handicapped in the mobile world, the blind in the seeing world, the deaf in the hearing world, a woman in a man's world, a black person in the white world: To what extent do you try to fit in and to what degree do you insist on your own standards, trying to exact understanding and change? The former divides you from yourself, the latter usually separates you even further from others.

As I got off the train that day in Chiusi and settled down to wait for my connection, a rare sense of peace settled over me. I recognized it as a phase in the cycle of acceptance and resistance that characterizes my experience of this disease. Tomorrow I might be pretending again not to have it, and in some ways that might even be necessary or good, but at that particular outpost the difference had provided me with a sameness, and I kissed my own pinprick scarred fingertips and waved them at the couple gliding away on the tracks.

Until we meet again, indeed. We will, in those moments of alien recognition that come in the most surprising times and places. And, then and there, we will be among the luckiest people on earth.

part two

Black Coffee,

Malted Milk Shakes,

and Snow

Coming Fast

Across the

Prairie

Bright, clear sky over a plain so wide that the rim of the heavens cut down on it around the entire horizon. . . . Bright, clear sky to-day, to-morrow, and for all time to come.

. . . And sun! And still more sun! It set the heavens afire every morning; it grew with the day to quivering, golden light—then softened into all the shades of red and purple as evening fell. . . . Pure colour everywhere. A gust of wind, sweeping across the plain, threw into life waves of yellow and blue and green. Now and then a dead black wave would race over the scene . . . a cloud's gliding shadow . . . now and then. . . .

—O. E. Rölvaag, *Giants in the Earth*

Closing shifts at Dino's were a necessary evil. Somebody had to do it, if the health department weren't to close the place down, and because working there was otherwise fun and profitable, and because we loved Mary, we did our turns at cleanup with a cheerful manic bravado, the jukebox turned up loud to drown out the vacuum cleaner and our already soiled aprons flapping in a frenzy of wiping, scrubbing, and scouring. As in all things, Mary had taught us the proper order, the most efficient procedures to use, and we all worked together in a tight choreography, the occasional touch to elbow or back all that was needed as we passed each other in the tight spaces of kitchen and counter and booth area. No one but the cook went near the grill, and when he went to empty the frying vat and clean the filters a loud and clear "Coming through!" would boom out over the music and clatter of dishes. For the briefest moment, we would flatten ourselves against the wall to make way, then would resume our three-dimensional work.

By the time we had finished, the stainless-steel hood gleamed; the iron-gray surface of the grill was smooth and even; the coffeepots sat in a shiny row after being swished full of a concoction of ice, cleanser, and Sprite then run through the dishwasher; the plates and plastic glasses stood in neat stacks; the salt and sugar shakers, the mustard and ketchup squeeze bottles were neatly filled and arranged on trays; the splatters and drips from the milk shake machine had been eradicated; the bright colors of the Formica tables and counter had been restored with a vinegar solution; all the debris of straw wrappers and stray french fries had been suctioned from the dark carpet; and the tiny, cold bathroom had been swabbed and sterilized. Even the heavy smell of grease would be veiled in the odor of vinegar and soap, though it would never leave our clothes. My housemate Rachel and I designated our "Dino's clothes," and once you wore something to work you never wore it anywhere else.

But we loved working there. On Saturday nights, between when our last customers would leave and the cleaning would begin in earnest, we took a breather, ate whatever we wanted for dinner, counted our tips, and clowned around as college kids will. One of our favorite traditions was "disco on the stools," a parody of the music that had recently swept the country like a plague. Rachel, fond of songs with a strong and happy beat for cleanup, often chose "We Are Family" and the like from the limited jukebox selection. The rest of us felt compelled to make fun of her taste and, sitting at the counter, eating our tuna sandwiches or burgers, slurping up our milk shakes, maybe even indulging in an onion ring or two, we would begin to twist back and forth on the rotating diner stools, trying to energize ourselves for the nasty work ahead after the long shift behind us. Eventually this developed into an all-out dance routine, the only rule being that you had to maintain some kind of contact with the stool at all times. Usually, this progressed to all three of us—the cook and two waitresses—standing on stools, spinning and lip-synching to songs we otherwise couldn't stand. It would last only for a minute or two, then we'd get back to work.

Almost everyone who worked at Dino's was devoted to Mary, the kindly, stubborn, and energetic woman who owned and ran the place. There were exceptions—a guy named Nick threatened to sue her after she refused to let him wait tables. Male waiters, she said, never worked out. She would hire both women and men as cooks, but only women as waitstaff. Controversy ensued among the network of students who worked at Dino's and those who were customers—almost everyone in a tiny college town—but the storm blew over. Mary sighed. She had suffered enough at the hands of the male half of the species, and even though her decree went down hard in a philosophical sense—we all thought that everyone should be treated the same and we could see this as sex discrimination—Mary always told us the truth. We simply believed her, and Nick was a pain in the ass, as we already knew from his ex-girlfriend and his housemates, who complained that he refused to donate more than ten dollars a week to the household food budget. Nick as waiter—the idea horrified us; he would be delivering a lecture on Marxist economics instead of sandwiches and then jealously eyeing our better tips. Besides, no one had ever protected a privilege for us females, our gender had never before been an advantage, and it was revelatory to occupy a sought-after position without having to be responsible for the unfairness of it.

Gladly, Mary took all the heat. She was, in more aspects than just gender politics, our touchstone with "real life." Divorced, with two teenage kids, she saved and studied long years, and during my senior year sold Dino's so that she could go to law school in the Twin Cities. After she left, Dino's became a dirty little diner; while she presided it was a place of sparkling good humor and practical caring. Her dreams and goals, and her stories of past travails, provided revelations of their own. It was about the only place around where townies mixed with both Carleton and St. Olaf people, and did so without resentment, and it was all because of Mary.

Especially after she sold out to a mean-spirited couple of gals who were universally hated for their cheapening and reorganizing of Dino's, people speculated about how the business had been profitable for Mary. Not a typical businessperson, she didn't even keep a tape in the cash register. The guest checks went on a spindle, and if someone wanted a receipt we made a second copy by hand—and that was how Mary did her books. In fact, we paid ourselves out of the cash register—at the end of each shift, you'd write on a blank guest check your name, date, hours worked at what job and rate, and a total amount, then you'd put it in the till, count out the money, and put the cash in your pocket. Two older women worked regular day shifts, but most of us students worked one shift a week for spending money.

On any given Saturday, Rachel and I would arrive for one of two shifts, ten to four or four to closing. Even at ten, Mary would already be dancing behind the counter, twirling on her feet, her slender hips rotating in her tight jeans, one hand pouring coffee, the other straightening and clearing, her laugh and chatter lighting up the old men waiting for their early lunches. Lonnie, the ubiquitous retarded citizen who Mary fed regularly in return for shoveling and sweeping, would nod his head and smack his lips in satisfaction over his favorite bacon cheeseburger, his work done for the day. The hiss of a burger on the grill and the burble of fries in the vat sounded almost sleepy, like a large, loud creature waking up for the onslaught of the Saturday rush, which would last from noon to eight or so, with a lull around three. As soon as we arrived, we added the sound of the coffee grinder—amazingly for those days, Mary bought whole beans—and the shift cook would chime in with the zing of the electric slicer.

Behind the counter, over the milk shake machine and the racks of plastic glasses, hung the mottoes of the place, which Mary would frequently point out to customers as eternal truths: "Moderation is for monks" and "Too much of a good thing is wonderful."

The food at Dino's testified to this attitude, each plate a monument to excess. Onion rings as big as donuts, submarine sandwiches two feet long and nine or ten inches high, thick milk shakes with enough chocolate syrup or malt to make the tongue take note, endless refills of steaming coffee. But Mary had a certain interest in quality as well, and bought only the best grades of meat and the freshest produce—huge Vidalia onions, fresh ground chuck for the burgers, good pumpernickel bread and light, airy sub sandwich rolls, spicy dill pickles, real cheeses, and the essential coffee beans. You might get insipid margarine on your toast around the corner at Fred's Ideal Café, but not at Dino's: real butter was the thing.

Dino's exuded all kinds of generosity. Not only did Mary trade a small amount of Lonnie's labor for endless meals, she also fed other needy people on the cheap, delivering leftover food to local charities and instructing us on a complicated system of lower charges for certain regular patrons. One of these, a traumatized Vietnam vet, would sit countless hours at the counter, snacking on freebies we put in front of him, rolling cigarettes, and pointing out that the butts lined up in the ashtray reminded him of the body bags stacked on the tarmac "over there." He never paid for more than a cup of coffee.

Mary showed just as much beneficence to us college kids. We were welcome to whatever we wanted to eat during our breaks and after our shifts, and, though no one ever took undue advantage, we ate well. I myself must have drunk gallons and gallons of the fresh milk delivered straight from the dairy in large cans that turned upside down in the dispenser. With my two long blond braids and my habit of downing glasses of the cold, white liquid, I soon acquired the nickname of "Milk Maid." I didn't mind—it was Minnesota, after all, and my roommate had informed me that although Minnesota was officially "the land of lakes" and Wisconsin was "the dairy state," Wisconsin actually had more lakes and Minnesota more dairy production. I became a permanent addict of good milk and cheese, malt in my shakes, and strong, strong coffee. All of these, I thought, were the tastes of an adult, and I enjoyed my sense of making my own choices, moving beyond parental influence.

Sometimes, vaguely, I was aware that there were unstated conflicts here with my diabetes. But these were the years when I pretended that diabetes didn't matter much, and I was greatly rewarded for such an attitude by compliments about how well I "handled" my disease. I had proven that I could go far away from home to college, that I could manage by myself, and that I was not to be defined by my illness. I took a shot once a day, and, with my blood sugars running generally high, I had few episodes of hypoglycemia. If every now and then I felt a bit sluggish I would reduce my food intake for a few days, and I exhibited few outward signs of any illness. At Dino's, however, the temptation to overeat loomed large, although I knew that for a diabetic too much of a good thing might be dangerous rather than wonderful. "Moderation," Rachel noted one day when talking me out of a milk shake, "is for monks and you diabetics."

Mary herself never once commented about my food choices, but she showed her awareness of my health in other ways. Once, when I had trimmed the edge off my little finger in the meat slicer, Mary cleaned and bandaged my hand with the utmost care and asked if I wanted to go to the emergency room. I looked at her, incredulous, and shook my head. Despite the blood, it seemed a small injury to me.

"Okay," she said, "but no dishwashing for you. The last thing you need is some massive diabetic-type infection in your finger." Immediately, she reprioritized our tasks to keep my hands away from the dirty water. There were no complaints, either.

Following her lead, the atmosphere at Dino's was so open about people's failures and limitations that my own problem never seemed to set me apart too much. Our difficulties, even the often trivial college-kid crises, were treated with respect and consideration. Mary kept a small bar hidden in the back on a high shelf and when one of us came in worried about a boyfriend or a girlfriend or a grade, she would ask us to name our poison, and after some moments of sympathy, we decided whether we could work or not. She never hesitated to let you go home if you just weren't up for it.

Not that we weren't already beginning to participate in the realm of adult problems, too. One of us might show up for work at Dino's with bruises across her neck and up and down her arms like footprints, compliments of her handsome boyfriend. For a while, I myself dated an alcoholic who was as indiscriminate about who he would have sex with as where he would throw up. Fed up and conflicted about their experiences, several young women fought eating disorders, discovered an appeal in bisexuality, and came to the political decision not to date men anymore. A black friend was hassled by members of the African-American student group because she hung around too much with whites. Another girl had a father who would send her nightmarish "care" packages; one day she received one containing a lovely roasted chicken—home-cooked, wrapped in aluminum foil, and now of course completely maggot-filled. One friend on campus was arrested for possession of speed and LSD, ruining her hopes of becoming a lawyer. Another acquaintance, caught sleeping with his girlfriend's roommate, had a nervous breakdown and was institutionalized; in his occasional calls from the psychiatric ward, he sounded as limp as a plant without water. We decided that *he* was definitely drugged, though legally. He never came back.

None of this ever surprised Mary, and she listened to our stories with equanimity and kindness, showing no undue prejudice or need to judge. What mattered to her was whether you could do your job, though she didn't punish you if you couldn't. Most of the time, upset or not, we came to work as scheduled. For us, work provided a simple task we could do well in good company, a comforting immersion in uncomplicated yet not unsophisticated values. Continuity, clarity, rhythm, teamwork, milk shakes, and subs provided relief from our web of social conflicts and our exposure to the likes of algorithms, Augustinian ethics, Lévi-Strauss's notions of the raw and the cooked, Giotto's gilded perspective, Zeno's never-arriving arrow, and the past historic tense of French verbs.

One deadly slow Saturday, the powdery snow falling steadily

through the Minnesota January afternoon, like a veil of sheets billowing in the twenty-below breeze, like a silent, white, stinging slap, as chill and bluish as the restaurant was yellow and warm, we hunkered down with our coffee cups for nonprofit boredom. Already, Rachel and I had reordered the stock shelves in the back room, cleaned out all the dishwasher filters, and scoured down every inch of stainless steel; Glenn had been on his hands and knees with a scrub brush and degreaser. We languished at the counter while Mary prowled back and forth in front of us, refilling our heavy brown coffee mugs and staring out the window into the weather. By three it seemed night had fallen, the snow brilliant against the darkening sky, but so thick that it sparkled only under the streetlights. Mary got on the phone to cancel the evening shift; we could stay an extra hour or so to serve the few bedraggled souls who staggered in, but not many would. At least, for the time being, we enjoyed our cozy camaraderie. Fortunately, the apartment that Rachel and I shared with two other women was just around the corner, above the shoe store. We could follow a wall all the way home, though Glenn would have more of a challenge getting back to his house a quarter-mile away and Mary, too, more than half a mile.

"I suppose I could always sleep upstairs"—Mary grinned at our concern—"but that would probably be worse for my health than passing out in a snowbank."

Over our mugs, Rachel and I exchanged a meaningful glance, our eyebrows rising in a tandem of surprise and mild self-reproach. How could we have never thought about what was upstairs at Dino's? We lived in an apartment on the second floor of this same block of crumbling old buildings in downtown Northfield, and such places, despite their usual crumminess, were coveted. How could Mary not be renting out her second floor?

"What's up there?" Rachel asked.

"Rooms," Mary said. "Junk. Dust." She hesitated, but then went on as if anticipating our thoughts. "I rented rooms for quite some time, but it was a pain in the ass. I'd finally had enough, and when another guy died, I threw everyone out and closed it down. Just shut the door." She snapped her fingers. "Like that."

"What did he die of?" I wanted to know.

"How many people died up there?" Rachel contributed.

"Is there any furniture left?" asked Glenn.

Mary laughed. "It was a little different then, as you students weren't allowed to live off-campus. I rented mostly to older people, like Lonnie, like Vic, and a lot of worthless scum. The whole thing depressed me." Her fingers fluttered in the air. "Half the time they didn't pay their rent, and they always squabbled about this or that, someone supposedly stealing somebody else's cigarettes or making too much noise coughing through the night, or someone would set the curtains on fire with a hot plate, or I'd come in and four pillows would have disappeared and . . . you can imagine. It was disgusting. I got tired of being a maid for those types."

We had never heard Mary say such judgmental things before, and though we appreciated her confidence in our student natures, we also knew that students could be horrible tenants. When we had taken over our place, we'd had to clean the debris out of one room with a shovel; we'd had to paint everything, use two bottles of bleach on the toilet and shower stall, and scrub the kitchen floor on hands and knees four times, each of us once. One paper plate, stuck to the wall with some oozing, sticky substance, remained underneath our new coat of paint.

Our furniture, scavenged from curbs, dumps, and secondhand stores or passed on from graduating seniors, leaked stuffing, squeaked, and sagged. The place was a dump, but we had traded decency for privacy, as we could each have our own room, and a kitchen where we could produce fabulous, non–dining hall meals. The $30 a month we each paid in rent was reasonable enough. Mr. Berg, the sweating fat man who ran the shoe store and was our landlord, said he would never rent to boys again. The place didn't look as if he cared at all, but he was pleased enough with our efforts to clean up that he offered to provide the paint.

"Most students wouldn't be any better," Rachel said, looking at me again with remembered disgust in her hazel eyes.

"Well, Northfield hasn't had too many of them die in their beds of alcohol poisoning," Mary said. "I hope that doesn't start happening anytime soon." I counted in my mind the number of alcoholics I knew who were my age: ten or twelve definite ones and that many more candidates. And these were just the ones I knew pretty well. How many of them will end up in stupors in dirty rooms? I wondered.

"Can we see?" Rachel propositioned. It would be like looking at the future—rooms once occupied now abandoned, their history revealed and concealed, traces left of people long gone from Northfield, as we knew we would be soon enough. Besides, Rachel and I were both studying sculpture and were on the constant lookout for interesting and usable objects to incorporate into our work. Maybe some expressive bauble would jump out at us from the trash.

Mary looked dubious, but the day had bored all of us silly, so she dug her ring of keys out of her ample purse and led us to the end of the hall near the restroom. The door screeched open to reveal several cartons of paper goods. "Gee, I must've stored this stuff here when the closet got full," she said as we clambered around the boxes into the stale, mote-penetrated air. "Don't open the door to the outside stairs. I'm sure they're rotten."

"Aren't you coming?" Glenn asked her.

Mary shook her head. "No way."

"It smells like rat poison," Rachel noted.

Indeed, little green pellets littered the floor, and we tried to avoid them like worms on the sidewalk after a rain, but the sounds differed, no sickening damp squishes but light, lifeless skitters and crunches with tiny echoes in what seemed a vast, dead space. And yet the long, narrow hall led us, and the doors, each left ajar at some unique angle, beckoned. The patched and dust-covered linoleum floor, floral in some places, flecked with brown dots or checks in others, creaked like an old man's knees as we stepped across it. Set at odd angles around the rooms, the beds and bureaus seemed frozen in motion, as if caught in some madcap dance by our entrance. Hanging from a bottom rung, a metal hanger clanked against the leg of a skinny chair. Our mouths and nostrils filled with powdery residue.

"It smells like abandonment," I said quietly to Rachel.

"Not to mention looks like it," she agreed.

"In more ways than one," Glenn added.

Everything seemed to be in the wrong place: ashtrays empty but coffee cups filled with butts; a bar of soap floating in the toilet; a roll of toilet paper on the coat rack; a suitcase sticking out of a chest of drawers in a room where hats, picture frames, and bottles of nail polish spilled across the closet floor. Yellowed newspapers and dirty magazines sprawled open in the corners. From every nook, booze bottles peered in arrogant defiance, all of them empty, soulless, and hard—graceful green wine bottles in one realm, square whiskies in another, a third fiefdom peopled only by harmless-looking miniatures, the certain off-spring of alcoholism, so Mary had told us. Now we knew how she knew.

On my one foray away from Rachel, I stood in a pale blue room with a floral linoleum floor at the end of the hallway, drawn to the brightness of the streetlight outside the window, barely visible through the dense wall of falling snow. This room, stripped cleaner than the others, seemed almost peaceful, cool and luminous as a prayer, and I drew closer to the window to see how far into the blizzard I could see—the sidewalk below, the store-fronts across the street, the traffic signal out on the highway? There, in the rim of the windowsill, perhaps once hidden by an addictor an old woman who feared the addicts, three orange-capped syringes cringed. The white outside the window appeared a solid mass and suddenly I felt suffocated, paralyzed, frozen, punctured, stabbed, and afraid. What was I doing here, so far from home? Would I ever live in a room like this? How can this happen to anyone? Then, next door, Glenn bumped into a chair, which screeched its protest, and I could move.

Quickly, the three of us retracted into a nervous knot, herded by the malevolent objects. We had all noticed that the beds were still made up, though unmade, with faded chenille bedspreads and hideous sheets twisted into corpselike piles over bare, rusty springs and sagging in the middle of peeling metal frames. Except one. Now we stood in the doorway facing it, yanked full into the middle of the room and with its fulsome mattress bared. Still showing a faded blue stripe around the edge, its lumpy flesh looked like a third-degree burn covered in Mary Kay face powder. The dusty but oozing brown stain leaked over the edge and pooled on the linoleum as tortured and alive-looking as if some-one had bled there yesterday.

"What'd you find?" Mary asked, back downstairs.

"Dust."

"Junk."

"Death," I whispered, awakening to my own condition, feeling more alive in this trembling awareness than I ever had before.

4

Hunger and Plenty

My first two years of college were a culinary void. Living as I did in Carleton's dorms, I ate in the dining halls where the institutional food was notoriously bland and disgusting. Even the apples and bananas didn't remain fresh, as they were cut in half in order to keep students from taking them back to our dorm rooms and stockpiling. During my unbearable two-week stint working in one of the food service kitchens, I received instruction on how to dip the cut ends in potato preservative to "retard browning," but this strategy merely created a toughened, slimy surface that had to be cut off again anyway. At meals we sighed and rolled our eyes, and smirked ruefully about having to eat retarded fruit. Still, other things were worse.

"What's for dinner tonight?" one might ask on the way in the door.

"Beige foam with tomato sauce," might be the reply. Or, "Beige foam with mixed vegetables."

Soon enough, however, we realized that the vegetables, too, tasted like beige foam. Thus, the beige foam theory took on shape and elaboration. *Everything* prepared, owned, and used by, everything remotely associated with the food service, run by Saga Corporation, had as its material base beige foam, even the Saga ladies, who worked in the kitchens and behind the counters in their uniforms and hairnets, sometimes cheerful but usually dour as they scooped the day's glop onto our plates. The Saga ladies were the most complex, additive-laden product, no doubt, but those food service types could make beige foam look like almost anything: lettuce with a sulfite flavor, hamburger charred almost black, thin brown coffee (thickened in terms of color, but thinned in terms of texture), chiffon fillings in "graham cracker" crusts. Even the silverware was really constituted of beige foam: fork tines commonly bent when faced with the tougher foam version of Saga mystery meat.

In those late-seventies years, vegetarianism had yet to take hold, and special dietary needs got about as much respect as Richard Nixon. As a diabetic in the dining hall, I shifted for myself, without knowing the ingredients or carbohydrate and fat content of the spaghetti and meat sauce, the cheese-coated cauliflower, the too-sweet corn muffins, the heavy salad dressing full of hidden sugar. Mostly, I ate just as everyone else did—impulsively, randomly, and with little thought about my health. Most of us, however, continued to long for the decent eats of home, the tradition of sitting around a table laden with a common meal to be shared, enjoyed, and digested into strength and energy. In retrospect, I imagine that Saga really wasn't all that bad, but at the time I hungered for home cooking.

Oh, for the chicken and dumplings, fluffy and hearty at the same time, savory in the light gravy with tender bits of meat seasoned with pepper. Oh, for the red, ripe tomatoes from the farmer's market, which we would eat like apples, trying to keep the juice from staining our shirts. Oh, for the simple omelet, onions and mushrooms peeking shyly from its edges. Oh, for the tartness of cranberry nut bread rendered even more piquant by my mother's blue cheese spread. I dreamed of all the good breads of home—whole wheat honey, banana, light buttermilk biscuits, refrigerator rolls, crusty cornbread not too sweet but ready to soak up the pot liquor from black-eyed peas or green beans. Oh, for ripe fruit, a rarity in Minnesota. I was horrified that people actually thought that pears were *supposed* to be crunchy, and peaches, too.

I was not alone in my dismay about dining hall fare, being a part of the last generation to be raised on family meals cooked at home, but also part of the new trend toward demanding individual accommodations. A group of students proposed, then organized, a vegetarian component for the dining halls. Based on a survey of students, they would receive a budget and a corner of one dining hall kitchen to prepare vegetarian entrees every evening. Student-cooked veggie, as it became known, grew so popular with vegetarians and meat-eaters alike that Saga soon ended the program. The scrumptious spinach lasagna and even the tasty soybean and vegetable casseroles simply made the institutional offerings look too bad.

Although a desire for privacy played a role, too, food was one of the main reasons I moved into an apartment my junior year of college. I needed to reclaim the healthy, food-loving attitude I had grown up with, to escape the quirky habits and compensatory nature of dorm dining hall eating. If I was going to obsess about food, as admittedly I did and still do, like so many females and so many diabetics, then I needed to have a sane space to do it in.

Things seem different nowadays. The undergraduates I know

who live in apartments don't cook; in fact, hardly anyone cooks anymore, even housewives. Accustomed from childhood to McDonald's and Hardee's, to ordering whatever they want at any given meal, to eating on no particular schedule and with no particular ritual, many students suffer no loss of continuity when they go to college and eat in dining halls. When they move into apartments, their eating stays basically the same: hamburgers and pizza, frozen Lean Cuisine in a plastic tray, instant macaroni and cheese. A few extreme fanatics pay attention to food, but often in a way that's joyless and compulsive, almost fetishistic, all about control or showing off, being superior. In my college days, in my particular milieu, food was still considered central to living well, a basic need and right. It nourished, fulfilled, satisfied, carried meaning and love, though of course it was never completely innocent.

Before my brother and I had a chance to become really picky, my parents had us bamboozled into believing that grownups, which at the time we still wanted to be, ate everything and loved it. Never forced to clean our plates, we were nonetheless required to "try" everything. But the main psychological strategy my parents used was simply to enjoy their food, and to make fun of us when we grimaced about broccoli or oysters or brussels sprouts.

"Someday," my mother would sigh, shaking her head in mock pity, "you'll understand. You'll figure out just how tasty corned beef and cabbage really is. When you're more mature."

Kelly and I would slant our eyes toward each other, suspicious but basically already conquered.

"I don't know if you'll like it," my father would say over his pizza layered in anchovies, at the same time looking longingly at its oily surface as though he coveted it beyond belief. "I don't want to waste it on someone who doesn't appreciate it."

Evenings in the kitchen my mother might give us the easy tasks—snapping green beans and brushing the silk off corn while the water already steamed in a boiling pot on the stove. While I played with the glistening golden strands, the flowing hair of the corn stalks, alternately pretending each one was my blond little baby and picking each one clean because I knew from experience how nasty cooked strands were between the teeth, Mom would hum along with the radio, her sharp knife flashing until rows of neatly sliced carrots and radish roses blossomed in neat piles on the cutting board. "Aren't they pretty?" she'd point out. Then she might tell the story of Rapunzel and the radishes, a magical, sought-after rarity that we could now buy at the grocery store any time we wanted.

The saliva would spring in our mouths, ready for almost anything.

My brother would sit at the table for hours on weekend mornings, so long that eventually the rest of us would give up and leave him there as we went about our day. Except my grandfather, and when he visited he sat till the very end, lending support to Kelly's methodical decimation of eggs, grits, biscuits, pancakes, whatever was the specialty of the day, marveling over a growing boy's ability to "put it away."

My grandfather, tall and fit his entire life, had long ago ceased to consume at such a rate, but he liked keeping up with our growth, and this certainly included the physical element, in rather quantifiable ways. Not only did he count my brother's biscuits, but he kept track of our height along the inside molding of a closet door at his house. Backing up against the doorframe was a ritual of our arrival for visits there. How many sit-ups can you do? How high a stick can you jump over? How far can you throw this baseball? Eating heartily signaled health and competitive drive.

He also showed us our way around a garden, taking us out to pick a few ears of corn for dinner, pinch the suckers off the tomato vines, and thump the watermelons as they neared ripe-ness. In these scenes, in the joy he took in our strength and vital-ity and that of plants, too, I came to understand the idea of plenty, of bounteousness. My grandfather passed on the sense that it was, indeed, miraculous that here lay this dirt, out of which, with the right care, would emerge these lush plants, which in turn would feed us and, in the correct balance, allow us to flourish.

"Where does all that food go?" he'd reflect as my brother ate. He provided us with the amazing answer: It turned into us and into our activities, into bone and motion. We thought that was pretty cool.

When Kelly slowed and seemed to be satiated, my grandfather would tell him to stand up and shake his long limbs.

"Pack it on down," he'd grin, "and you'll be able to fit a little more into those hollow legs."

If my brother was the champion of food consumption, however, my goal as female and diabetic gradually turned into being the champion of restraint, of walking the fine line between not enough and too much. There is no need for me to rehearse com-mentary about our culture's emphasis on thinness for females, but medical instruction, interacting with that culture, makes diabetic girls absolutely ripe for eating disorders. Even a recent American Diabetes Association booklet on diet gives as its top two of three "nutritional goals of diabetes management": "appropriate blood-glucose and blood-fat levels" and "reasonable weight," never noting that for us Type 1's these two goals are often in direct conflict. Tight control for us brings weight gain. In fact, the average weight gain after the initiation of treatment for Type 1 diabetes is about ten pounds, a trauma for girls who have no doubt been praised and envied for their overly thin diabetic bodies. A body that can't move sugar into cells, as insulin allows it to do, simply excretes that sugar and all the calories that would otherwise accumulate if the body could use them. Even if I had not had a doctor who put me on a 3,000-calorie diet at diagnosis, I surely would have gained some weight.

Many diabetic teenage girls take to skipping injections as a way of losing the extra pounds. That may increase their chances of being blind in fifteen years, or of dying of a heart attack by age forty-five, or of spending years on kidney dialysis, losing their legs to gangrene, having uncontrollable bowels and bladder, or being incapacitated by a stroke, but, hey, that will be later. Even next week, they are likely to end up in the hospital from ketoacidosis, the poisoning that comes when the body breaks itself down for energy to run on. Teenage girls are at the highest risk of diabetic coma of any segment of the diabetic population. But, in the moment, they, like almost all of us women and girls, want to be willowy, tiny, as light as a breeze, and they are willing to suffer otherwise to be so.

"Compliance" with treatment plans is what the medical establishment seeks to inculcate, not eating disorders, but standard treatments for diabetes I believe also breed anorexic and binge-purge habits. Anorexia, it has long been acknowledged, is at least partially about control. One of my college friends, the daughter of a housewife and a rather severe Presbyterian minister, had a sister with a classic case of anorexia. She described dinners in that household looming every evening like the Salem witch trials, powerful father in black presiding over a table where he considered it the moral responsibility of everyone there to eat what God had provided, where all the girls were quizzed about their activities and results of school tests, where attendance and clean plates were required, no disagreement or discussion tolerated. My friend's sister simply quit eating. She proved her point about who was in control of her body.

At age eleven, just when I began to exercise some decision-making power about my life, control over what I ate was similarly taken away. I faced all kinds of rules and regs about what I "could" and "couldn't" eat, in precisely what quantities I must eat, and at what times I must and must not eat. It's not even as simple as just avoiding concentrated sweets. Rather, the diabetic must achieve a careful balance of carbohydrate and insulin intake. Nowadays I use a method called "carbohydrate counting," wherein I can estimate the number of carbohydrate grams in *any* desired combination of foods and take a variable amount of insulin calculated to match. But in the old days, and still often today, with an unvarying prescribed dosage of insulin came a traditional meal plan from which you were never to stray. The diabetic exchange diet, doubtless developed in order to make eating simple for the afflicted, consists of milk, meat, bread, fruit, fat, and vegetable "exchange lists," and it is only within those parameters that you are allowed to vary your diet.

For breakfast you might be told to eat one bread, one meat, one milk, one fruit, and one fat, which could translate into a piece of toast with a teaspoon of butter or margarine, one egg (not cooked in additional fat if you're going to butter your toast), one cup of milk, and a half cup of orange juice. Tomorrow you might have low-sugar cereal with some sliced strawberries and milk, and some stray dish of cottage cheese (cheeses count as meats, not milks), but, by golly, you've got to have fruit every morning.

This obsessive measuring and counting, the hyperawareness the lists show of fat content of foods, and the rule-laden way of eating that completely disallows certain ingredients are all reminiscent of the compulsive patterns of anorexia and bulimia. None of it has anything to do with what you're hungry for, or, in fact, whether you're hungry at all.

Hunger, for me, became a confusing sign. In a diabetic it may signal low blood sugar—when the body is depleted of food, hypoglycemia is more likely—but it can also accompany high blood sugar—if the body is not using the food it is consuming, it starves. Later, when many of my college friends were trying to recover from sick eating habits, "eating only when you're hungry" became the popular measure of health, but at best I could only make that an ideal set aside whenever my blood sugar fell.

And, when the blood glucose has fallen far enough to make me shake and perspire and grow mildly incoherent, I get frightened. I find myself half out of my mind with hypoglycemia, quivering like a bowl of Jell-O and only dimly perceiving my situation, instinctively going to the refrigerator for juice or the cabinet for glucose tablets. Yet it is in that very moment that I need to be self-controlled, to eat only three tablets or to drink only half a cup of orange juice and then wait calmly for fifteen minutes to see if I feel better. If not, then eat more, but not until then. An unreal proposition. My instinct is to eat ravenously until I feel better. But that is often a mistake and I overdo it, eating so much that my blood sugar is set upon a roller coaster. If you eat too much when your blood sugar is low, in an hour or two it may swing too high. Then the corrective measure of extra insulin, if not carefully timed and calculated, can send you crashing to the bottom again, and a vicious cycle ensues.

There are also larger, longer swings, entire days when my blood sugar just seems to stay high, no matter how much insulin I take or how little food I eat, other days when it crashes repeatedly, even though I've eaten candy bar after candy bar. This can be influenced by many factors—other illnesses such as viruses or even mild infections (the latter of which we diabetics have a hard time fighting off and which I, for one, carry almost all the time); stress; a skipped exercise session, or an extra one, or even one that just varies a bit from the usual; any variations in the speed of your digestive tract on a given day; and another aspect of food, called the glycemic index. The glycemic index refers to the speed at which something is usually digested. It isn't only *how much* carbohydrate something contains, but *how quickly* it will enter your bloodstream. But different people, at different times and under different circumstances, digest different foods at different rates.

Last night, for instance, I ate a large Greek salad for dinner: two cups of lettuce, a quarter of a tomato, a slice of onion, a sixth of a green pepper, about three ounces of feta cheese, eight or ten Greek olives, a tablespoon of olive oil, and some vinegar. Along with it, I ate two modest slices of whole wheat, unsweetened French-type bread. How did I match my insulin dosage? Well, as my doctor has calculated it, I need 1 unit of insulin for every 10 grams of carbs I eat—and I am lucky for this easy-to-multiply even number, as opposed to those who need 1 unit for, say every 8 or 12 grams. I also add or subtract units depending on a sliding scale of what my actual blood sugar is. So, before last night's dinner, when my blood sugar tested in at 181 mg/dl, I calculated my dosage as follows: 6 units to cover my meal (two cups of raw vegetables and two "bread exchanges," or approximately 60 grams of carbohydrates) and 1 unit extra because my blood glucose was on the high side, for a total of 7 units. In fact, I knew that I was shorting a little, as my sliding scale for adjusting my insulin dosage indicated I should take 2 extra units, but I hesitate to take too much extra in the evening as I don't want to go low when I'm asleep. I'd rather have the bgs stay up at 150 or 180, even 200.

However, by bedtime, my blood sugar rang in at 340. Huh? Granted, I hadn't had any exercise the day before—I'd been on jury duty—and I'd gotten upset over a conflict with someone doing work on my apartment in the late afternoon, but 340?! Was this caused by the lack of exercise? The anger? Was my insulin too old and getting weak? Had the insulin spoiled from the heat on this first sultry day of June? Maybe my body wasn't absorbing the insulin and it was just sitting under my skin waiting for more activity in order to work (more circulatory action also goes with more exercise). Or was it the bagel I had eaten for lunch—lots of carbohydrates with a fairly low glycemic index—finally kicking in? Or was it a sign of developing gastroparesis, a relatively common side effect of diabetic nerve damage that causes the stomach to empty too slowly and/or unpredictably? What could I do about it anyway? I took 4 more units of insulin, something I hardly ever do at bedtime, but my blood sugar remained over 300 when I got up this morning. Again, I adjusted my dosage with my sliding scale and ate my usual breakfast. By noon, it had risen to 421. Unbelievable. And frustrating.

I go through this kind of thought process every time I eat, or if I don't I should. How I answer all those questions determines what I should do to correct my blood sugar, though my calculations don't always work out. But notice the similarity between these calculations and the fearful negotiations that anorexics go through every time they eat. Diabetics are given an eating disorder as part of a prescription for survival. If we let it go too far, we, like anorexics and bulimics, will hurt ourselves, but to some degree our unnatural obsessions about eating are necessary.

I myself have never skipped injections intentionally, though I've occasionally forgotten them when caught up in other things. Perhaps I would have skipped shots during my teenage years if I'd thought of it as a method of weight control—certainly I have worried about my weight continually since I turned twelve—but I never did. I had very limited exposure to other diabetic kids, and perhaps that had its advantages: no whispered strategies for fooling the 'rents and the docs. True, too, that standards for control weren't as tight when I was growing up, and, so, even though I took my shots, I didn't know the level of my blood sugar and therefore could never track the relationship between my control and my weight. My weight fluctuated pretty widely. I didn't really understand that much about why.

My rebellion took the form of eating whatever I wanted. Most of the time this didn't involve anything too extreme—I'd nibble the occasional cookie or chomp down a small bag of popcorn at the movies with my friends, but my mother had applied herself diligently and enthusiastically to making my diabetic diet palatable, and so I was mostly satisfied with meals at home.

I'm from a family of wonderful cooks, long lines on both sides of the family tree, and my mother is no exception. Southern women, of course, have a reputation for this, and in my experience it's a stereotype that's also true. In my little wooden recipe box, I still carry the instructions for my Great-Grandmother Craddock's steam-cooked cornbread, a rather sweet version you cook in a double boiler over a pot of beans, and in a corner of my kitchen counter sits, ready, my Great-Grandmother Roney's blue bowl and her hand-crank coffee grinder, which still works even though she used it every day of her career as a farmer's wife. My Grandmother Meek had majored in home economics in her college days and had taught it briefly before dedicating herself to her own family duties, and her own daughter, my mother, though she went on to earn degrees and have a career in education, also got her bachelor's in home ec.

Perhaps this turn to academics in the realm of food rendered my mother open to change, for when the doctors lectured my parents on the need for alterations in the standard southern diet for someone with diabetes, my mother easily rose to the occasion. It was out with the fried chicken and in with baked chicken and rice, out with overcooked green beans with bacon and in with al dente snow peas, out with pecan pie and in with fresh fruit and yogurt. My diabetes changed the entire family's diet for the better, nutritionally; both of my father's parents and my mother's mother grew heavy with age, but neither of my parents has developed any significant problem with weight, and my brother has remained thin as a beanpole all these years.

But cravings for fat and sugar seem to be either hard-wired into us or such a site of cultural longing that they are impossible to resist completely. The expectation that someone should resist them completely leads rather directly to the binge-purge mentality of bulimia, and I have certainly been no exception to that. In fact, I know hardly anyone, and especially not any woman, who doesn't participate in this kind of overeating followed by some type of self-punishment, whether it be fasting for a day or two, cycling onto a severe diet, running three (or ten) miles, or simply brow-beating oneself for being fat—all short of anorexia and bulimia, but nonetheless cut from the same cloth. We are terrified of being overweight, not to mention the fact that overeating is simply physically painful, yet for some reason we long to cram our mouths full. And do. You would think we would stop, that it would be the kind of thing like touching a flame—you do it once and you learn that it hurts, makes you feel gross, so you don't do it again, at least not for a long time. While there are obviously only a few who become obsessed with pain in a variety of masochistic ways, nothing is more culturally common than hurting ourselves with food (well, there's alcohol . . .).

It's all a matter of degree, too. In response to the mottoes on the wall at Dino's, I developed my own: "Too much of a good thing is wonderful, every now and then" and "Live immoderately—in moderation." But I've continued to wonder. Why do people hurt themselves so much both by overeating and by hating themselves for even an occasional food indulgence?

I had a secretary once who worried a lot about her weight. A borderline Type 2 diabetic and continually on and off restricted diets and exercise plans—always outrageously difficult so that her failure was guaranteed—she fulminated at her desk daily about her sins, whining that she hadn't lost any pounds, promising to do better, mumbling derogatory terms at herself. One warm, hectic day, in a whirl of thirst and overwork, making a quick side trip for a soda to the dark back hall where the vending machines were, I came upon this woman standing in the shadowy corner, cramming a candy bar down her throat.

One hand covering the lower half of her face, she hastened to throw the wrapper into the trash can and gulped the remainder of the chocolate down barely chewed. Her eyes looked startled, hurt, frantic, like a cornered cat.

I plunked my change into the soda machine, punched for a Diet Pepsi, and waited as it thunked heavily into the slot.

"Oh, my God," she began, finally swallowing the last, her consonants still sticking on the syrupy thickness in her mouth, "you caught me."

"Eating a candy bar," I interrupted, "is not a crime. I didn't catch you because you're not doing anything wrong. It really isn't a moral issue to eat a little chocolate."

I was harsh. I was abrupt. I did not comfort her or sympathize openly. Clearly, she wanted to go on, to make excuses or to castigate herself, but I couldn't listen. This particular woman drove the entire office crazy hating herself so openly. Most of us either balanced it with more positive feelings or at least hid it better. Then, too, I had been there myself too many times: secret eating, hating myself for loving the taste of chocolate, wanting to appear invulnerable to greed and desire.

"Eat another one, if it makes you happy," I said as I departed. "But for God's sake, bring it to your desk and enjoy it." I left her standing beside the vending machines, marched back to my desk with my soda, and never mentioned it again. There was, in fact, no need to marvel: almost all of us have been in that same spot.

At the end of my junior year in college, on my way to a summer internship in Washington, I stopped in New Jersey to visit my uncle and his family—a fairly unfamiliar part of my family, with some measure of hostility between my uncle's wife and my grandparents and parents. I went because my uncle, an amateur watercolorist, wanted to take me to the Picasso exhibit at the Museum of Modern Art, the first ever of the mega museum shows. Wound up tight as a cuckoo clock, having just cut off all my long hair and on my way to my first big-city adventure, uncomfortable with my aunt's sneering judgments, I tried to remain on absolutely "good" diabetic dietary behavior. I don't remember the specific dishes we ate at meals, but I do remember them as rather bland and stringent, things like unadorned rather dry pork roast and boiled, saltless green beans, and I recall my aunt's admonition as she served her husband and daughter their ice cream for dessert, her eyes as cool and blanched as her own lime sherbert: "Would you like an apple, since you're not allowed to have sweets?" I felt fat, childish, and controlled.

One afternoon my aunt announced that she needed to run out for a few errands—would I be okay on my own until my cousin Mary got home from high school? The tidy, empty house echoed the unvarying tick of the kitchen clock, and the drone of a lawn mower in the distance seemed to well up in the living room as solid as the clouds over Picasso's *Blue Roofs* of Paris. For the first time in days, my lungs relaxed, my spine loosened, and I lay my head against the back of the chair and rocked, thinking about the fragmented faces of Fernande, Marie-Thérèse, Dora, Françoise, and Jacqueline, and the more traditional portraits of Olga, the wife.

Suddenly, before my eyes, Picasso's creamy whites turned into vanilla, his glossy browns into chocolate and cinnamon, the bright purples and reds of the thirties paintings into fruit flavors. The cheeks of Dora Maar turned into strawberry, her tunic into boysenberry, while Fernande swirled in a fudge ripple. I just had to have some of that ice cream tucked away in the refrigerator, forbidden to me.

In one swoop I moved to the kitchen and stood in front of the open freezer, carton in hand. Already guilty, but beckoned by the icy weight in my grasp, I decided to dispense with a bowl—I would only take a bite and for that I needed only a spoon, which I soon enough located in the drawer by the sink. Furtively, I edged into the living room because from there, through the imperious floor-to-ceiling windows, I could see the driveway and any imminent approach from the street. One bite, of course, turned into two, then three, and, even though my mind was blotted and dulled by the inimical sweetness on my tongue, I worried that the calculator eyes of my aunt might detect the missing spoonfuls, so I snapped the lid down. Stop, I thought. Enough.

At that moment, too late, I heard my cousin's key, the kitchen door opening, and the footsteps coming across the floor. In a panic, I thrust the ice-cream box underneath the sofa where I perched. Surely, I thought, she'll pass on and dump her stuff in her bedroom. Then I'll have my chance.

"In here," I called out.

Mary paused in the archway and tried to look friendly, but all I could think about was the ice cream melting in its cardboard on the wan carpeting under the furniture. How long did I have?

"I was looking out the windows," I explained to Mary's question-mark expression. Clearly, the living room was seldom used except when my aunt played the piano. Mary nodded, turned, and went back through the hall and into the kitchen.

"Gotta start my homework," she informed me.

Doesn't she even need to pee? I wondered. Doesn't she even want to change clothes? But Mary went into the kitchen, poured herself something to drink, and set about laying out her books on the table. I knew that I had to get the ice cream back into the freezer. Now. Mary's impassive stare would not be as bad as my aunt's flinty squint and pressed lips, and the latter would be home any minute. Besides, the ice cream must be getting squishier, more liquid by the minute, and soon my predicament would bring irrevocable damage. So, flushing in shame, I retrieved it from its warm coffin under the couch, checked for leaks with my palm on the rug, and marched back into the kitchen. Mary turned slightly and watched me replace the carton in the freezer.

"I was cheating," I said.

She only nodded and returned her gaze to the pages in front of her nose, which wrinkled slightly with what I was certain was disgust.

Predictably, my disordered habits of eating started in childhood with a longing for the sweets forbidden to diabetics. It didn't take long to figure out that if I wanted to sneak a candy bar, the effects on my urine sugar would be less obvious if I also skipped my lunch. The common term—then and now—for a diabetic's eating of sweets is "cheating," and I became a cheater, just like the lowest kids in school, who copied off other students' exams and tried not to get caught. My parents fortunately had sense enough that around our house there were also a certain number of sanctioned "treats," comprising the occasional half cup of vanilla ice cream or the one-inch square of angel food cake. Still, I also cheated.

In retrospect, I think this had to do mostly with fitting in, not making a big deal about one more difference that separated me from other kids my age. I had always been a little odd and had always suffered terribly from feelings of rejection. But fitting in and not making a big deal about my diabetes was also the attitude that was medically and socially sanctioned beyond the world of peer pressure. How could I be expected to simultaneously fit in and behave so differently that I didn't eat with my friends?

In high school, playing cards every few nights with Kelly and our friends Jay and Ruthie, I might sacrifice regular Coke for Tab, but that wasn't noticeable once they were poured into glasses. Potato chips were a different matter.

In cahoots with my friend Susan, the cheating sometimes became real bingeing. Most often, this happened at her house where I'd go for a sleepover and her parents would retire early, leaving us the TV in the den and the larder stocked with all kinds of goodies, available in infinite quantities—unlike at my house, where I was aware of a quiet surveillance of the pantry, almost sneakier than any eating I might do. As Susan's family was one that still regularly had the traditional full-course meals, there might also be leftover desserts—caramel cake, apple or lemon meringue pie, brownies, fudge—lined up along the counter on glass-covered cake plates, ready at hand. We would settle in front of the luminous flicker of the tube, the surrounding room darkened, our bowls of ice cream and packages of cookies arrayed around us, our pajamas loose and comfortable. Volume on the television turned low, just enough noise to screen our secret conversations and the rustle of cellophane packages, we would embark on long nights of gossip and food. Though the next day we would refer to ourselves as "Thunder Thighs" and "Beached Whale," we would eat with abandon, sickening ourselves for reasons that remain mysterious.

By the time I went away to college, my secret eating binges were a habit well ensconced. Never particularly severe, they still brought me fifteen or so extra pounds and a great deal of shame. I am not a secretive person, nor am I one who bears up well under physical pain, so my days as a binger were, from the beginning, I think, limited. Already, I had begun refusing to attend the popular Sunday brunches at the Hyatt Regency Hotel in Knoxville, where my friends, male and female alike, loved to go and pay the then large sum of twelve or fifteen dollars to gorge themselves on unlimited omelets, crepes, croissants, strawberry cheesecake, fresh-squeezed orange juice, and champagne. I just couldn't bear to eat that much at one sitting and I hated the atmosphere of gluttony: the hiss and smoke of too much butter sizzling in the omelet and crepe pans; the well-dressed after-church crowd milling from serving table to serving table, filling and refilling their plates, ogling the trays of meats, cheeses, sweet rolls, and fruit; the embarrassed side glances that evaluated who could eat the most while appearing moderate. I suppose it has always been easier for me to confront myself in other people's behavior, to see how it should be altered in *them*. I knew those people should cease eating so much, just as I knew years later that my secretary should quit harassing herself for eating at all, but I could not find the balance myself.

Getting out of the dorms and dining halls, which I did my junior year at Carleton, marked the beginning of my return to mostly healthy attitudes about food, saner eating habits, less in the way of self-castigation. Partly, this resulted from feminist and lesbian consciousness-raising. Two of my roommates that year were bisexual, one lesbian, and all were older than I. The apartment brimmed with feminist publications explaining breast self-exams and menstrual sponges and echoed with conversations about the tyranny of the fashion industry, the unfairness of beauty standards, and how we could heal the brutal damage we all felt had been done to us by our male-dominated society. By the end of the school year, I had shed my long, blond locks for a short butch haircut, even though I didn't have a lesbian bone in my body. The hair had been a lot of trouble, and it represented my male-pleasing desperate vanity, so it had to go.

Rachel, who struggled with her own food issues, and I clung to the feminist literature on weight and eating, like hummingbirds to the scarlet feeder—it offered sustenance and hope, but we fluttered in and out because habits are hard to change. One horribly titled but wonderful little self-help book, *Fat Is a Feminist Issue*, by Susie Orbach, gave us our most helpful tip from that pile of literature: forgive yourself if you slip up. In a context where we forgave each other, that became almost possible.

But the simpler thing that turned around my eating attitudes even more than feminism was that my apartment mates and I channeled our food obsessions into a different pattern, working at the food co-op, planning elaborate meals for one another, sampling a variety of international cuisines. Instead of competing over who could eat the most (or the least), we vied over who could cook the most creative meals, who could go the longest without repeating a menu or dish, who could please everyone's palate at the dinner table. This provided a fabulous release from the cycle of overeating and fearing and hating food. Once more, it became a source of joy and pleasure.

Shaun moved into the apartment a few weeks after Rachel, Julie, and I had settled in, a new recruit to replace a woman who had decided not to come back to school. We needed her to make ends meet, but she made me nervous, as I knew that she and Julie were becoming involved, and Shaun approached this change in her sexuality with her typical over-the-top enthusiasm. She also had a lot of stuff. Up the long, creaky staircase to the second-floor apartment, banging through the door repeatedly, we hauled Shaun's heavy possessions that in themselves brought an air of permanence to her presence. Into the kitchen went her twenty-five-pound drum of special rice, her cumbersome cast-iron soup pot, the wok that would not fit into the already crowded cabinets, a knife block full of cleavers. Into the racks went a panoply of little cellophane packages full of dried mushrooms and transparent noodles, sticky bottles of strange vinegars and dark sauces, and tubes of brown pastes lettered in foreign alphabets. Worst of all, into the refrigerator went a cracked plastic tub of a vile-smelling, shiny, black goo she told us was miso. Soon pushed to the back corner, it sat squat and forbidding, traces of its stench creeping out to remind us of the unknown.

As Irish as she was in name and background, Shaun was a devotee of Asian cuisines. She had lived for a year with a Chinese-American family and had thoroughly adopted their eating habits, later adding Japanese and Thai elements to her repertoire. Proudly she noted that she hardly ever ate with knife and fork anymore. "If I can't eat it with chopsticks," she said, "I'm just not interested." Soup was the main exception, and Shaun boasted a lovely collection of porcelain bowls and Chinese soup spoons, which she used with ice cream, too. Everything else she ate with her fingers or chopsticks—quiche, strawberries and cream, steamed spinach, polenta, Rachel's dolmas, Julie's hand-cut ravioli, my ratatouille. Though I considered this habit pretentious, I could not complain when Shaun set out to feed us.

Anyone who insisted on buying a particular variety of rice in massive quantities would have to be reckoned with. Shaun explained that in Chinese and Japanese culture, rice is the meal, that the rest is extra. She noted that while the miso seemed disgusting in concentrated form, a tiny bit of it could add pungent flavor to a variety of dishes, that it carried an almost magical reputation for promoting health and beneficence. She was eager to participate in our round-robin ritual of preparing dinners for each other, and soon her meals would become the expected highlight of the week.

She had won me over the very first time she made us a meal at our apartment overlooking Northfield's Bridge Square, harking back, as I think she did, to my parents and their attitude of mysterious superiority over unfamiliar foods. In the strangest of ways, she both reconnected me to my childhood sense of the goodness of food and expanded that sense to include a fascination with the variety of tastes and textures available around the world. Once more a kid, I hung around the doorway of the kitchen, watching as she shredded scallions, roll-chopped carrots, and set tofu to marinating in soy sauce and ginger.

That first Shaun meal, a Chinese-Japanese amalgam that would horrify any purist, steamed out of the kitchen into the dining and living room with all the presence of a dragon. As Shaun had chopped and stirred in preparation, we had sipped hot sake from tiny green mugs until we flushed and groaned with hunger. Then Shaun retreated back into the kitchen, and the sizzle of vegetables in the wok tantalized us momentarily before the stir-fry and fragrant jasmine rice appeared in a flurry in front of us— hot and satisfying on this cool Minnesota evening, but fresh and green and crunchy, with no sign of the dead winter to come. We emulated Shaun, picking up one little piece at a time with her precise chopsticks, enjoying both the common sauce and the individual colors and flavors of the vegetables, laughing and chattering at the slow, gentle progress of our eating in spite of our ravenous appetites.

But it was the miso soup, served next, that filled the room with its strong steam. I sat looking down into the thin brown liquid, a few shiitakes and carrots bobbing aimlessly, the bright green of the chopped scallions luridly floating on top, and wondered how on earth such a weak-looking soup could fill the room with such a rich smell. Then I remembered the evil carton in the refrigerator. Momentarily, my stomach churned. Did I really want to taste this stuff?

Julie looked as uncertain as I did; Rachel, more urbane,

already waved her spoon nonchalantly; Shaun slanted her eyes to the side as if to emphasize that this was not a test, she was not watching us, she did not care whether or not we liked the soup. Of course, we did.

It was not that I put an end to all my conflicts over food then—during my junior year. Witness my New Jersey ice-cream escapades. The next year, too, I had a roommate fond of the Scarsdale Diet, and every so often all six of us would go on the diet together, although none of us was seriously overweight. This posed some problems for both my newfound sense of my body as something I shouldn't punish and for my diabetes, but I did it nonetheless. Everyone understood that if my blood sugar got low, I had to eat "off the Scarsdale," but that rarely happened, as my blood sugars ran generally high during that period. I would worry obsessively about my weight for the next six or seven years, and would never cease completely to worry about it.

But in that year I began to understand the complexity of the food matrix and to be able to hold on to the pleasure possible in that particular bodily process even in the face of its many abuses.

I think of the champagne brunches my senior-year roommates and I threw, replete with homemade goodies, all day eating and drinking, loud music, marijuana in the later hours, and congenial contributions made by even those who came uninvited—and these parties were famous enough that people did crash them. Ah, the cinnamon rolls, the pistachio bread, the apricot cake, the chiles rellenos, the deviled eggs with spicy Hungarian paprika, the tabouli, Greek potato salad, eggs Benedict, the blueberry crepes, the café au lait. This occasional indulgence allowed me to be calmer the rest of the time, my continued impulses toward excess funneled into these few but magnificent events. And, even there, such a sense of never-ending plenty filled the room that none of us felt it necessary to gobble.

I think of living with Julia in St. Paul, the year after I graduated, the coldest Minnesota winter in forty-five years, struggling, unhappy, uncertain what direction to take, but nonetheless certain that there would be homemade muffins for breakfast and thick, puddinglike hot chocolate to cast off the evening chill, to fortify me against the job-hunting rejections and the loneliness of a strange city. Both of us broke, yet creative, Julia and I made portrait cookies of our friends for their Christmas presents, cutting them out with kitchen knives, then decorating them with a palette of colored frostings we'd mixed ourselves. One cookie per friend is not much of a gift, but their likenesses were so accurate that they were a big success.

I think of cooking a southern dinner for my dear friend and picky eater Charlene, her sister-in-law, that woman's boyfriend, who was from my hometown, and a college student I'd been doing some work with. Nothing unusual about this, except that I was extremely self-conscious of my whiteness and all of their blackness. Another student (white) had not been able to come, and I found myself in the position of being a "dumb white girl" cooking for the demanding taste of a couple of black southerners. I have never seen anyone, not even my brother as a teenager, eat so many country ham biscuits as Roxy's friend did that night. We laughed and laughed at his respite from homesickness about food, and, to my delight and Charlene's horror at his forwardness, he even asked for some to take home with him when he left.

. . .

I think of my seduction via food by my lover Panos, a temperamental Greek man, who impressed me with his ability and willingness to cook.

"What can I do to help?" I'd ask as he prepared dinner in his apartment filled with satin-upholstered carved antiques, Ming vases left by his dead mother, his grandmother's oil portrait hanging over the dining table.

"Adorn the furniture," he'd joke, as he checked the leg of lamb, the lemon chicken, the olive oil–roasted potatoes, the spanikopita, the artichokes awaiting their Hollandaise sauce, or the pungent Greek salad and dusty bakery bread ready to sop up the lemon-garlic dressing and stray bits of onion.

He almost always washed all the dishes, and he was faithful as the sun about timing meals consistent with my diabetic regimen. He even cooked me an octopus, once upon a time. Is it any wonder that I loved him?

Food times aren't always so happy. I think of another lover, caught out as a philanderer after I had sublet my apartment and traveled three thousand miles to spend the summer with him. Both of us normally fairly ascetic eaters, creatures of habit and health, we could hardly stand each other as we waited for the summer to end so that I could go home. The tension at our shared meals made the usual salads and bagels difficult to chew, much less digest. In fact, I began to have fairly frequent hypoglycemic episodes due to my failing appetite and so began to keep sweet, crunchy, easily digestible cookies around the house. Gradually, we began to try to find all the varieties of Pepperidge Farm cookies—they were the best and we were going to rank them all. We developed a scoring system based on three qualities—appearance, taste, and texture—and careened all over town from grocery store to gourmet shop to find every possible variety. It gave us something neutral to talk about, even though we often disagreed about the merits of particular cookies. Nauseated at Bill's deceit and perversion, I survived the rest of the summer on cookies and yogurt, which was about all I could keep down. It might not have been the greatest strategy for a diabetic, but I managed to get through the summer without killing him— or myself.

Eating is a process that never ends, and for the diabetic eating is a regimen, a routine, a more or less cast-iron plan for every day. I get tired of it, wish for days when I could just sleep straight through without eating, long for a chocolate malted without guilt and complex calculations to try to balance out the sugar with extra insulin, wonder what it would be like to choose something completely unknown off a menu. Still, as constrained as I feel by the diabetic rules, I have broken many of them in the interest of a different form of health, to escape the eating-disordered thinking that comes with such a proscriptive concern with food. To move back and forth between eating like a diabetic and eating like a "normal" person is the key for me, prevents me from hating the digestive process that keeps us all, even diabetics, alive.

Recently, in a diabetes e-mail discussion forum a member recounted the story of taking his young diabetic daughter to the fair, where other children munched on popcorn, slurped snow cones and lemonade, and feasted on ice cream and cotton candy. The man, eliciting sympathy, mentioned the sad look on his little girl's face when he made her understand that she could never have such things. As did several others, I posted an immediate response: Get real. You may be able to control your daughter completely now, but what you need to be teaching her for her teen and adult years is how to indulge—occasionally and responsibly. Otherwise you will be inducing in her such self-hatred and guilt that she will never recover. One man, a diabetic for something like three decades, with excellent levels of blood sugar control, announced that at least three times a year he allowed himself a "hog-wild" day, where, though he tried to adjust his insulin accordingly, he let himself eat whatever he pleased. All of this was lost on the well-intentioned father, and he replied that he will keep his daughter's blood sugar as tightly reined as possible so that she will still be complication-free when a cure is someday found.

What this man misses is that neurosis is a complication, too. Even if his daughter doesn't turn his vigilance into her own diabetic anorexia, she likely will suffer feelings of marginalization that he can't imagine. Would that eating were a mere bodily function, but it comprises a complex social matrix, and we all need to participate in it in order to be part of the group.

Eating alone, as I do so often now, bores me and often leads me to eat poorly even though the diabetic regimen should ostensibly be simpler without the complications of others' preferences and schedules. I still prefer to share meals, and my favorite one to make for a group of guests is an antipasto with a ring loaf of salty, sesame seed–covered bread or garlic and rosemary focaccia right out of the oven. The bread, in preparation half the day, breathing and rising, shaped so intimately by my fingers and palms, and filling the house with its clean, honest odor, anchors a table covered in large platters and small dishes. A bowl of piquant leaf lettuce and arugula; piles of tomato, onion, and green pepper slices; hard salami and prosciutto in paper-thin slivers; creamy chunks of fresh mozzarella with chopped fresh basil; spicy marinated eggplant; artichoke hearts; wrinkled Greek olives; and jars of balsamic vinegar and golden olive oil stand ready. If it's a big occasion, this course will be followed by a mass of spaghetti or fettuccine and a couple of easy sauces—pesto and tomato with orange juice or tomato-onion and creamy Gorgonzola for the rich at heart. No one ever wants dessert.

We all gather around the table, crowding in, jostling and touching elbows and hands as we pass the numerous serving dishes and transfer food to our plates. Usually at this meal no one really eats all that much. The Chianti or Rioja flows, the conversation is always free and animated, and selecting and arranging the food—handing the olives to Anthony, making sure that Danielle gets some mozzarella, that Jim and Rick remember the necessary dash of dark vinegar—becomes more important than shoveling it into one's mouth. The meal is a site for connection, and it always takes me back to my grandparents' blue kitchen, where we would cram into the corner for the hungry talk and I had never heard of diabetes.

5

Running in Place

I stood at the edge of the pool, my toes gripping the concrete like desperate little hands, their skin pressed into the gritty surface by my metatarsal bones and my skeleton of inflexible fear. In contrast to my mood, the water slapped at the edges, cute, as persistent and frolicsome as a three-year-old tugging at my sleeve. Light flickered through the cavernous space, flitting over faces and bodies, sparkling in the drops of water flung from fingers and hair, dancing on top of the liquid without a care in the world. And the sounds themselves rocked gently against the walls, muted and soothing; the air billowed against my face, warm and humid, peaceful and friendly as the quintessential womb.

Not comforted, I quivered to the bone with cold, my usual sense of alienation heightened by the calm surroundings. I waited my turn to try to pass the swimming test required for graduation from Carleton. Probably I would succeed, as I had spent the past few weeks in a swimming class, not having had the nerve to try the test when administered the first week of classes. Instead, I had signed right up for a swimming course and, twice a week for nine weeks, had been floundering around in the pool with a bunch of other uncoordinated slobs.

I looked down at my body. It felt gray and small, but looked pale pink and large, an abalone where I expected a shaking bit of seaweed. My navy blue tank suit seemed wrapped around cotton candy, as empty as an erased chalkboard, a long tunnel under the mountain with the lights off, a black hole expanding in space. From its edges, however, bulged my thighs, solid, firm, massive as Stonehenge boulders, though gooseflesh mottled their surface. I could see a drop hanging in my eyelash, could see the rim of my cheek, the angle of my elbows, but under all this flesh what I felt was my skeleton, brittle and afraid, and my heart slamming against the bones from the inside. And cold, I felt cold.

About the time the instructor told me my turn had arrived, I realized my blood sugar was low.

Unable to conceive of how to straighten out the tangle if I interrupted the smooth flow of the testing process, unable to break out of the rhythm, I dove anyway—an awkward, stiff plunge in which my shins nearly scraped the pool's edge. My toes did not want to let go of the concrete, but I told myself that the instructor wouldn't let me drown, so it'd be worth the risk to go ahead and get the whole thing over with.

Suddenly there I was, moving through the water, my limbs functioning almost smoothly. Now, in the pool, I could feel the buoy of my flesh, the effort of my muscles, the swell of lungs. All term I'd been working on this automatic adjustment to becoming a creature of the sea. The water held me; all I had to do was breathe and pull my arms and flutter my feet. Easy enough, I thought, although my coordination was off and my mouth kept filling with water I had to swallow. Still, I was gliding through the green, muffled in this comfortable fluid, not needing to think.

Then I nearly rammed my head into the wall. I had forgotten it would be there, which in itself was shocking and embarrassing, but I had also failed to see it right there in front of me. At the last second, I shot up out of the water, gulped air, and pushed myself weakly back toward the other end. So much for the fancy under-water turns I had been trying to perfect in the past couple of weeks—I could not bring myself to try them, as I now envisioned myself confused by the upside-down whirl, diving in the wrong direction, flailing toward the bottom of the pool. I reverted to the clumsy reach, the slow sideways turn with head above water, and the twisted kick behind. At least I didn't forget the wall again, and I completed my hundred yards before dragging myself up out of the pool. The instructor's disappointed look faded as I panted about my blood sugar.

"Inelegant," she smiled, handing me a towel, "but you proba-bly won't drown."

She turned to the next student, and I scurried off for the locker room, my wallet, and a sugared soda from the machine. For such a lousy swimmer, teeth chattering in hypoglycemic hypothermia, I felt ridiculously triumphant.

I've had to face it. I will never be a good swimmer. In fact, I will never be any kind of very good athlete. Not ever. I dream of win-ning some sweepstakes that would allow me to live unimpeded, to train four or five hours a day, to grow steely and tanned. But I know that won't happen. My body has already been the best it will ever be. By the time we are thirty, this is true for most of us; with diabetes, the downhill direction is even harder to slow. It is no wonder, then, that it can be so difficult to continue to struggle, to feel that the effort of exercise is worth anything. Oriented as we are to the values of endless economic growth, to progress and self-improvement, how on earth are we to find this futile activity satisfying? As a diabetic, already overwhelmed with the maintenance of my body, the filing of health insurance claims, and a low energy level, why on earth would I want to take on the further complications of rigorous exercise?

Without a doubt, I can say: Because it's the only thing that makes a noticeable difference in the way I feel. Exercise, I've found, is the closest thing there is to a key to happiness and well-being. It's that simple.

It's not, of course, that insulin doesn't make me feel good, but I experience that only in its absence, as feeling ill. When my insulin levels are on target, granted I feel comparatively better than when they are high or low, but that feels *normal*. The same may be said for a host of other factors in the diabetic equation. When I eat too much, I feel sick. When I don't sleep well, I get a headache. When I drink too much, I pay for it the next day. Exercise affects the other side of the equation. I don't feel bad when I skip it, though sometimes I get sluggish or antsy; it's just that I feel great when I do it.

Sometimes I think this adds to the difficulties of maintaining an exercise program. When you don't eat, your body eventually cries out for food. If you get tired enough, you drop into sleep wherever you are. But it's the external environment that by design calls us to activity, and we just don't live that way in our society anymore. We sit at desks, drive machines, stroll for our food through the aisles of an air-conditioned grocery store, effort-lessly pushing a cart on wheels. We are not very often chased by enemies that might eat us, nor do we chase our dinner, and the body does not cry out when we don't stretch and move it. It only, eventually, sags.

This sagging, of course, kills more people than gunshot wounds, and as a nation we are incredibly out of shape. My mother refers to the Virginia city where she lives as "the land of the fat people," but you see the grossly obese wherever you go, in every average American town. What I notice is that, as in so many other ways, there seems to be a growing divide between the haves and the have-nots. The middle class shrinks, the rich get richer, the poor get poorer. People eat either in the fanciest nouvelle cuisine restaurants, where tiny slices of organically grown vegetables are garnished by a swirl of sweet potato puree for $24.50 or they eat grease-laden fries for $1.50 at McDonald's. At the malls the overweight rest on benches every fifteen minutes, but the gyms and health clubs are crammed with hard bodies pumping iron for hours every day.

I myself have never wanted either to court death or to pretend it would never capture me; both extremes feel like denial to me, or perhaps it's just that I'm too vain for the one, too lazy for the other. At any rate, when I turned twenty-eight, and my butt began to hang below my underwear line, I decided I had to join the gym even though I was not the type. I knew I would never accomplish the standard look, would never proudly parade between the Nautilus machines in skintight pink spandex, hardened midriff exposed and biceps bulging, my face made up and my hair neatly tied into a bouncy ponytail on top of my head. I didn't really even aspire to that. I just wanted to feel a little firmer.

Charlene and I braved the weight room at Rec Hall one day after work. We stopped at the sign-in desk to show our IDs and make an appointment to learn how to use the weight and stair machines, but that day we had to be satisfied with spending a few minutes pedaling away on the stationary bikes. No one was hostile, exactly, but an air of dismissiveness surrounded us. Lined with mirrors, the room seemed to reflect our ignorance, our uncertainty, our lack of muscle. We pedaled and talked office politics, and Charlene beamed her charming smile at every person who passed. "Hi," she'd say in her heavy Georgia accent. "How long have you been working out?"

Everyone clearly thought us crazy or pathetic or both.

"Do you want to keep doing this?" she asked as we walked to our cars afterward, our gym bags dangling from our shoulders with our briefcases, our sweat-dampened clothes chilling in the fall air.

"Yes," I said. "I'm tired of letting the assholes have everything."

We were there twice a week for two years, and we even made a few friends among the muscled crowd thanks to Charlene's continued charm. Much to our relief, our personalities did not change, but we both grew stronger and experienced that fabulous sense of blood flowing through warm and supple tissue, our very own bodies, not ones we saw on TV. There with my fledgling pecs and abs, I felt as powerful as any mega-athlete, because this accomplishment, no matter how small, was mine.

Walking is still my favorite physical activity. If I had all the time in the world and a series of available trails, I would spend half of every day walking. One of my favorite things about living a small-town academic lifestyle is that I walk all the time: to and from home and campus, back and forth to the library, across campus to teach a class, downtown to meet a colleague for coffee, by the credit union to deposit a check, into the drugstore to pick up my insulin and syringes. A friend of mine bought me an old bicycle and tried to convince me that it was more efficient to get around that way. I missed my own stride too much, and I was always forgetting the combination to the lock. So, while I still use it sometimes, I've mostly gone back to walking. I go to the gym, play the occasional game of squash, do some yoga when feeling stiff, but what I really like to do is to walk. I feel as though I could walk across the country.

I stood in the early evening light flickering through the half-grown spring leaves on the arching limbs high above me. I knew, as my grandfather had taught me, that these were forest-grown trees, their long trunks reaching for the scarce light, unlike those trees planted alone, which spread wide like umbrellas. My brown peanut of a dog, Not Spot, stretched and scratched idly beside me, waiting for Mom, occasionally sniffing the mild breeze, her black eyes still a bit somber and sleepy.

"Do you want to go for a walk?" I teased her, and she jumped, prodding me with her toenails, her jaws widening into a distinct grin, her black-mottled, part-Chow tongue extending ever so slightly. I uncoiled the hose, turned the squeaky spigot handle, and pointed the spray over the impatiens under the front window. Notty nipped at the stream as if it were a leash and she could pull me along.

By the time my mother emerged from the house, the flowers merely dripped, the hose lay neatly wound, and Tacky and O.J., our monstrous old cats, had joined me and the dog on the driveway. We had our entourage. While Mom, Notty, and I would walk at least a mile, the cats would come merely to the turn-around of our dead-end street and back to the house, then we'd go on down the hill and around the corner, leaving them to their cat business. Still, I loved that sensation of walking and chatting with my mother, examining the trillium or the blackberries along the way, accompanied by the ever joyous dog, with the two cats trailing along companionably, shy O.J. lurking in the bushes, Tacky meandering down the middle of the street, placing his huge killer paws gently, almost primly, on the pavement, his magnificent black tail waving in the air.

That air itself was as important as the companionship. The air in the native forests of East Tennessee has an extraordinary quality most of the time—a piney fragrance, just the right level of humidity and coolness, a smooth, clean feel against your skin. You can't help taking deep, almost gulping breaths when you step into that air—your nostrils fill with it and your lungs fill with it and they want more, more. Even my tired diabetic body always felt refreshed and ready to stride off into that air.

Of course, even after I had careened to the ground from the back of my mare when I was eleven, I also loved riding horses; I still do when I get the occasional chance. I kept a horse until I went to college, when my parents made it clear that I couldn't both keep the horse *and* go away to school. I chose the education, but to this day I know the precise pattern of how a horse's hair grows; the way it splits into two directions at the joint of the hip; how it coarsens from the hock to the fetlock; and where the softest parts are, both the obvious ones, like the nose, and those often overlooked, like the dip where the neck joins the chest. Still, I dream about the sensation of communicating with the powerful, nervous body of a horse, of indicating a turn with a leg-squeeze, of calling a huge animal to a halt by merely closing my fingers, and also of letting go of the reins, trusting a horse to clamber up a rocky hillside unguided, allowing him to race the other ponies across a pasture, of charging whooping and free through the tall grass.

In some ways, walking and horseback riding couldn't be more different activities. One of them can be done almost anywhere under almost any circumstances with no requirements for special equipment (unless you consider a decent pair of shoes special).

The other takes a stable, pastureland, fences, rings and jumps, oats or sweet feed, hay, a farrier, saddles, bridles, halters, lead lines, saddle soap, Lexol, buckets, brushes, hoof picks, immunizations and veterinarians, trailers, trainers, boots, hard hats, and assorted other basic necessities, including the horse itself, which takes many extra hours of care besides riding. Whereas walking is cheap and can be done by almost anyone, horseback riding is terribly expensive and requires skill and lessons.

But both of them are things you usually do outside, mall walking notwithstanding. For me there is something important about exercising outdoors, and this has to do with a sense of connectedness that I don't often feel. Even the physical activity itself, the motion and the respiration, the taking in of the outside air, the moving through a living space, grounds me in a way that seldom happens indoors, and never in an athletic facility. The landscape of the horses' bodies is part of the larger landscape across which we ride—and walk—and it's an environment in which I feel that I belong.

Maybe it's simply that I walked and rode before I became a diabetic. Consciously, I can't even remember anymore what it was like not to have this condition that splits me so from myself. I watch myself constantly, but outside it is easier to turn my eyes to what's external to me, and at the same time to feel part of it. A hawk circles high overhead. What kind is it? What is it hunting, or is its circling less intent today? Does it have hatchlings to feed? When it dips down, I see the rusty hue of its spreading fan of feathers: a red-tail, a fine raptor, living in suburbia, compromised, in danger, alone, going about the tasks of its daily existence over and over and over again, playing a role in relation to all other creatures, eating some, feeding others, perhaps wondering if it wouldn't be easier to be a wren or a sparrow. But it is a hawk.

Walking, I watch that solitary hawk, the chattering wrens and sparrows, the manic swallows, the rare bluebirds, the lumbering groundhog and spastic squirrels, and the unfurling leaves of grass and trees. Is a tree alone? Do leaves really whisper to each other, to me? At least, they breathe and, moving, I breathe with them. Sitting with binoculars is not the same; I cannot be merely a spectator. Instead, I must be going on about my business, the activity of supporting my own life, in a way that also allows me time to look around, to note my place among other living things.

There is so much to see in such small, repetitive places, where all change really occurs, and it's an odd thing to try to explain how this is connected to my body, the only one I'll ever get, the one that stays the same and changes all at once. The state of the weather seems comparable to my blood sugar levels—some days it makes exercise outdoors impossible, but most of the time it is just something to take into consideration. Underneath my feet runs the same old trail; in my veins, the same old blood. And yet the path discloses one day worms wriggling in the tempting warm rain; on another their darkening, drying alphabet-shaped corpses, sometimes covered in ant specks; a day or two later, the asphalt is as black and clean as a newly washed chalkboard. Over the years, my body will not only observe, but follow this same trajectory. Even day to day my heartbeat varies, sometimes my legs hurt, or I feel groggy with glucose imbalance. Some people lose interest staying in one place for very long, but I never get bored as long as I can walk, experiencing my own change and the daily drama of tiny lives and deaths.

Riding requires lots of time and money; even strolling for fitness takes a lot of time. While I still use the latter as my main means of transportation to work and back, I don't have the hours to walk enough to stay in shape. So, I also jog. In my own head I call it running, but once a man at my gym asked me how far I go, and when I replied he said, "You don't run. You jog." Whatever.

It's slow. I don't go great distances. But I think of it as running nonetheless, and it has been a virtual constant in my life for the past ten years. The guy who corrected my terminology may be able to go out and push himself to run ten miles, but he was chubby enough that I suspect he's someone who only occasionally goes out and hurts himself. None of these weekend warriors looks particularly great, but they are always ready to put you in your place if you are a moderate exerciser like myself. My mother, I want to tell them, never took up a sport in her life— never ran, played tennis, never stuck with aerobics more than a few weeks—and she's in better shape for her age than anyone else I know. She just walked all the time, slow, steady, no stress. Still does.

I don't believe in suffering any more pain than necessary, and I know from experience that if I push myself too hard I will quit exercising to avoid the pain. My philosophy, over the years, has gradually become "Too little, very often." Even though I've known a couple of diabetics who were in great physical shape, much better than I am, I think that the forgiving attitude is an absolute necessity for those of us who exercise. Too many of us are trying to be the athletes we'll never be, and we suffer needlessly, we fail to get any exercise out of shame for not being able to get a lot.

Diabetes complicates exercise quite a bit, in several different ways, and so for many years we diabetics were not really encouraged to exercise, at least not we insulin-dependent types. First of all, exercise increases the risks of hypoglycemia, as happened to me during my college swimming test. The most obvious risk for diabetics in general, hypoglycemia becomes downright frequent for diabetics during intense exercise.

Just yesterday, I went for an ordinary late-morning run that I couldn't complete due to low blood sugar. This doesn't happen to me often, as I almost always test my blood sugar before strenuous exercise, but it slipped my mind that I'd had a couple of glasses of beer the evening before, and alcohol, over a period of up to twenty-four hours (usually about twelve to eighteen for me) lowers blood sugar, sometimes dramatically. I had a normal blood sugar of 125 before I lifted a few arm weights, then drank a full glass of grape juice before heading out for the bike trail. Fortunately, I also carried with me a full tube of fast-acting glucose tablets, as is my habit, because about a mile and a half from home I experienced that familiar old sensation of dragging feet, accelerated heartbeat, and shaky fatigue. Every stride became a terror—would I fall? was I getting so confused I might be in danger? would my heart burst?—and yet I tried to choke down a few glucose tabs as I continued to try to run. Finally, I walked for five minutes, ate *all* the tablets I had, and then alternated jogging five minutes and walking five minutes until I got home.

Why did I keep going? The expert advice on exercise for diabetics is, like so much medicalized information, technically apt but real-life difficult if not impossible. One book I have suggests that you stop and test your blood sugar every 15 to 30 minutes during a workout and, if you encounter a low, to stop exercising, eat a snack, wait 15 minutes, then test again before resuming your activity. All of this advice is just fine—as long as you don't have anything else to do in your life. If I followed these guidelines, I think I'd give up before I got out the door.

Granted, I virtually always carry glucose tablets, and if my blood sugar gets low enough I stop and walk, but think about the real impact of this advice. Yesterday, I was a mile and a half from home, not even halfway through my standard workout. To turn around and walk home would have meant not only that I wouldn't get my full workout, but that it would take me almost twice as long. Frankly, I didn't have the time. I have also tried running with a fanny pack to carry my glucose meter, and that's as uncomfortable as wearing high-heeled shoes. I ended up with a raw spot scraped into my skin from the shifting and rubbing of the nylon bag. And, am I really supposed to stop out on the bike trail, in the wind or drizzle, whip out my beeping meter, and then sit around and wait fifteen minutes while my blood sugar rises back into completely normal range? I mean, I run all year-round. Sometimes it's 22 degrees out there. Even at the gym, on the treadmill or stair machine, I have to sign up for a specific time slot of twenty or thirty minutes; if I get off, I lose my turn. And I don't have time to reschedule and wait, reschedule and wait, reschedule and wait.

Sometimes I feel guilty about the way I flirt with this advice. Hypoglycemia is dangerous, and I have no desire to get so incoherent out on the trail that I pass out in someone's backyard or in a stand of trees behind the elementary school. But diabetes provides enough real reasons not to exercise, to put it off, to hold back, to "only walk" today, that it's really hard to know when to keep going and when to back off. As with all aspects of diabetes, it's a matter of balancing between the dictates of the illness and doing what you want to do; only with exercise, because most of us tend to be lazy, what you want to do for your health is often not what you want to do at the moment anyway. It's so easy to put it off that sometimes I probably overcompensate by pushing the limits when my blood sugar is on the low side.

The other end of the spectrum, by the way, is even worse, though not as immediately dangerous as hypos. Strenuous exercise with hyperglycemia—high blood sugar—also can be harmful, though, of course, for different reasons. A blood sugar of over 300 makes exercise impossible, as your body interprets it as stress and the blood sugar will rise even higher, instead of lowering as it normally does with physical activity. The healthy response to exercise is for the body to maintain a small amount of insulin in the bloodstream, for the liver to release glucose to fuel the muscles, which that minor amount of insulin then allows to be used. In a person with higher than normal blood sugar, however, the liver continues to release glucose, yet there is no insulin that allows the muscles to use it. Instead, the glucose level continues to rise in the blood, and, even worse, the waste products of the liver's conversion of fat cells into glucose—ketones—also begin to build up in the blood, causing it to become dangerously acidic. The body begins to poison itself.

Whether the blood sugar is high or low, however, the muscles aren't getting what they need to work. For this reason, diabetics often have difficulty achieving a training response in the muscles. With high blood sugar, in particular, lactic acid tends to build up, causing severe pain in the tissue. Fluctuations in blood sugar can also cause swings in the muscle content of sodium, calcium, and potassium, leading to frequent cramping and stiffness not due to muscle trauma. I get agonizing cramps in my feet at least once a week. It is, in general, difficult to improve, to strengthen, to condition—as difficult, it sometimes seems, as flying. The idea is there, the willingness and longing, too, but the body has its limitations.

All of these parameters and hindrances, I've found, make it difficult to retain exercise partners, that thing which all the advice books say you must have. Of course, because of the dangers of hypoglycemia, exercising alone has its risks. Though I occasionally enjoy a walk or run or session at the gym with a friend, on a day-to-day basis I prefer the control and simplicity of the solitary endeavor.

A few years ago, I started running with a friend of mine, a woman I'd already known for some time and to whom I had grown increasingly close. Rose claimed she would be a perfect exercise partner for the health-challenged me: misdiagnosed with a mild heart condition as an adolescent, she'd never been fit, though she was thin. She would be eternally grateful if I introduced her to the pleasures of regular exercise, and at first she was, though it did not last.

We ran together for the better part of two years, at first according to my old habits. Charlene had moved away, but I continued to work out with the weights and stair machine at the gym twice a week, and to run another three or four days. This routine, which I have now reestablished, worked well for me. It gave me some variation, but enough consistency that it didn't pose too many diabetic problems. I could swap the indoor workout for the outdoor on days when the weather was just too awful, and those days on the stair machine rested my shins, which was important as I'd had a tendency toward shin splints when I was younger. The weights improved my muscle tone and added to my strength, so I'd been able to finally increase my running times. I was in the second-best shape of my life, and for a graduate student that's saying something.

Gradually, however, my partnership with Rose eroded that situation—in tiny little steps, bit by teensy bit, Rose took control of my exercise program and inculcated in me an ugly shame about the "excuse" provided by my diabetes. I'm sure she never intended for this to happen, but it did. It took almost four months after I'd realized it for me to quit exercising with her; our friendship also came to an end, though there were other factors involved in that as well. Rose didn't like going to the gym—said that she couldn't get the hang of the stair machine and that the leg press made her back hurt—so, although I still tried to fit it in every now and then I basically gave it up. Instead, we ran nearly every day, and during that first winter we ran a lot on the indoor track, because Rose protested running outside if conditions were the least bit cold, damp, or icy. Even with the overheated, oxygen-depleted air of the indoor track, I convinced myself that it wasn't so bad as long as I had Rose to chat with as we jogged our endless circles.

During the next summer, however, Rose took more and more to changing our exercise times. I often had to sacrifice the ideals of diabetic exercise routine to other aspects of my life, so it seemed unfair to expect her to stick steadfastly to any schedule that I laid out. Although it troubled me that she frequently canceled evening appointments because she was "too tired," when she had insisted on those time slots in the first place and when that meant that I either couldn't go myself (for I don't run outdoors alone at night) or I'd have to go to the damn indoor track alone, I nonetheless just considered these occasions unfortunate coincidences.

She, however, developed the habit of questioning me when I canceled. My blood sugars must have seemed to her like a flimsy excuse, and she made no bones about rolling her eyes when I told her that I could only walk, that my blood glucose was 310, or 278, or whatever. Although she often called a halt to our jogging before I was ready to stop, she took to describing to me how much longer and faster were her few runs without me.

Then one day I found myself running along the crowded indoor track, elbowed by college students, my ankle complaining of the unrelenting upward curve of the floor, all alone at an inconvenient time. Rose was supposed to meet me at 5:15, after the class she taught, but when she hadn't arrived by 5:30, I'd begun without her, at first just stretching against the concrete block walls, swinging my arms and legs, doing a few sit-ups. Then I'd walked a couple of laps and started a slow jog, watching for her silhouette in the doorways all around. When she finally arrived, I waved, but she turned her back, sat down on the bleachers, and began changing into her running shoes.

She was furious, and when I paused so she could join me, she let me have it. What did it mean that I had started without her? Just that she was nearly half an hour late, I noted, and I had other things to do that evening. Was I saying that my time was more important than hers? No, I began to bristle, but when people habitually keep me waiting long amounts of time, I think they don't value mine. Besides, I said, *I am a diabetic*, and I have to get home and eat dinner on time. I *can't* just wait around. Implicitly she accused me of being jealous that her students wanted to talk with her after class, that her husband would be preparing dinner for her, that her main life's work was taking care of her daughter rather than pursuing a "stupid" Ph.D.

We smoothed it over, we ran around and around the track that night, we laughed, we apologized, both of us. But the next day, I happened to notice in the departmental directory that Rose had office hours scheduled at the same time she'd said she'd meet me at the track. All semester she had double-scheduled those minutes, had no doubt often hurried students through their questions, but had even more often kept me waiting idly until she arrived. My diabetes and the struggles it posed for me, I realized, meant little to her.

The day after I discovered Rose's deceit, I began to take my exercise program back into my own hands. These days, I often go for long walks with Carolyn, Leslee, or Holly. When Mark and I visit Craig and John in New York, he and I take a companionable jog around the reservoir in Central Park. And sometimes, I corner Mark for an inept though fun game of squash. As far as the regular, daily practice, however, I find the birds plenty of company. They do not compare my prowess with their own or point out my painful limitations.

Psychiatrist Arthur Kleinmann, in his book *The Illness Narratives*, recounts the story of a diabetic woman, depressed because painful peripheral neuropathy had forced her to give up her walks. She had fought this for years, and told her doctor when he tried to cheer her that her life was just shutting down bit by bit. He admitted that he could not deny the truth in that. I myself cringed and worried for weeks after reading this story, thinking of the joys of respiration and movement, of fresh air against my face, of my own sweat trickling down my back, of how I might lose my calm entirely if I did not have the reassurance of that simple embodied experience, even though I will never be a competitive athlete, even though my standards are necessarily low.

Like everyone, I hope that my end will not come in an agonizing, bit-by-bit decline, but as a diabetic I am far more likely to experience such a gradual diminishment. In some small ways, I experience it already. I try to accept that, to find in it something that I can look forward to learning, but I admit that I dread the prospect of not being able to meander long hours on pathways under trees with the bright red flame of the cardinal or the quick flash of the goldfinch keeping me company in the warm midday light, my breath and blood rising and dropping with the hills. I hope instead that a sudden heart attack leaves me lying on that ground, my running shoes on, my eyes turned toward the fluttering leaves above, undiscovered until darkness falls.

6

Living Off the Looming Darkness

Saturday morning, and I sat at the light table in the silk screen studio, alone in a building totally abandoned by others for college weekend pleasures. I had nibbled some granola and yogurt and left my roommates all still asleep to come and work on my secret project. Someone had told me not to do something, and so of course I was doing just that. The rebellious act of becoming an art major had not proved enough, and my confidence in the role had grown so that I could apply it to itself.

The silk screen print I labored over, tracing out shapes and cutting stencils over the hot light table, was a study in black. Mr. Warnholtz, my printmaking professor, had forbidden us to use black ink. "Black," he said, "is always made out of other colors. Make your own." But one innocent day, digging around in the cabinet full of ink cans, I had come across a tiny, corroded one labeled "black." The temptation was just too much. I promised myself that it would be an extra print, over the number required for the course, so that he couldn't count it against me, and I had shelled out my hard-earned money for additional sheets of the expensive but fabulously smooth Rives printing paper. These I divided by four, so that it only took me two sheets of paper to run an edition of eight small prints. I worked on them only at night or on weekends, so that Mr. Warnholtz would not forbid me to finish them, and I hid them in the far recesses of my assigned drawer in the studio. No one had seen them.

Mr. Warnholtz was also a big fan of transparent base, a see-through additive to be used with any color of ink. We didn't make silk screens like the ones you so often see in the commercial world or on T-shirts—the colors in hard-edged, opaque shapes that never overlap. Ours were studies in color interaction, one layer built onto others, the transparency that we stirred into the inks allowing for a depth and richness not often seen in the medium. We mixed a lot of inks in a lot of versions, constantly bringing in orange juice cans in which to whip up our own concoctions with the scrap wood Mr. Warnholtz cut into stir sticks and lidding them with the squares of scrap mat board that he also supplied. That way the inks didn't dry out and someone else could use them or adapt them once again. Although the inks and solvents were highly toxic, and I often left with a headache, the studio was a harmonious working space, well laid out, and suffused with the pleasant rhythm of cutting a stencil, mixing the right color, securing a screen in the hinges, setting out the stack of prints, laying each one in turn under the raised screen, turning on the vacuum to hold the paper in place, lowering the screen, scraping the ink across with a swish and a clunk, raising the screen, and removing each print to the drying rack. We moved peacefully around one another, sun streaming through the tall windows, our aprons splattered in riots of color, the noise of the vacuums creating an effective privacy, a cushioned sort of camaraderie.

I loved working in that room, and so I wondered at my own impulse to risk the wrath of Mr. Warnholtz and ruin it all. Mr. Warnholtz was the senior member of the art department faculty, and he had been around forever. He had built the vacuum tables we used, the drying racks, and the light table itself. In an old station wagon, some years before any of us students were born, he had driven hither and yon collecting the lithography stones that filled his handmade racks in another studio downstairs. I didn't even realize then how much better all his custom-made furniture was than any I would later encounter in commercially furnished studios. His designs made the place work, and nothing ever broke.

At the time, however, I was aware only that he was an old man and was moody. He was notoriously difficult to read, unpredictable, temperamental. All of our other teachers we called by first names, but in spite of his jeans and T-shirts we addressed him as Mr. Warnholtz. The source of much fear—he sometimes actually ordered people out of "his" studios, permanently—he expected the obedience and respect due his knowledge and experience. There was no doubt that he knew his stuff about prints, but some days, as he slouched against the counter along the back of the room, his unkempt white hair and teeth stained yellow from his constant smoking and his thick and spattered glasses sliding down his crooked nose, his gnarled fingers would begin to wave through the air and his lecture would slide from the technique of glue stencils to some garbled anecdotes that made no sense to any of us. On those days, we would sigh and whisper that he'd been breathing the poisonous solvent fumes too long.

So I had worked myself up into an entirely justifiable nervousness. There was, I knew, no telling how Mr. Warnholtz would react to my disobedience, and this risk rendered my activity all the more exciting.

In retrospect, I have grown to understand that my perhaps innately rebellious temperament combined with a physical cowardice (or, maybe, good sense) that grew out of the fearsome consequences of diabetes made me an intellectual daredevil instead of a million-other-kinds-of-risk-taker. Always restless, but without enough physical confidence to dance wildly or to drink until I passed out or to get up in front of crowds and lead the rallying cry against apartheid, I asserted my radical desires more quietly, trying to push the limits of my mind in the game of my schoolwork. I had to get my thrills somehow.

This is, I believe, part of what attracted me to the study of art in the first place. No doubt that innovation drives the machine of many professions, but it takes longer to earn the right to participate in it when you study math, science, history, psychology, even philosophy, which I had almost declared as my major my sophomore year. Instead, I turned straight into the realm that held the bohemian up for praise, where eccentricity was cultivated at least in theory, and where the limits hovered close enough that I could begin stretching them immediately. As a draftsman and painter I never showed much talent, but I always overflowed with ideas. By the time I took Mr. Warnholtz's printmaking class, I had already begun my senior project—a series of mixed-media sculptures of a narrative sort, made out of mostly discarded objects: books, boots, cardboard boxes, chairs, cigarette packages, maps, sequins, tennis balls, window frames with broken panes of glass. Of course, this wasn't completely new in the world of art, but it was new to me and felt like a realm in which I could do anything, go anywhere, escape all limitations.

How could anyone forbid me the black ink?

Before that Saturday, I had already laid down six or seven versions of black, with more or less transparent base, with bits of blue commingled with one, globs of yellow and green stirred into another, all of them mixing on the paper into what I was beginning to find a very rich and compelling darkness in a vaguely architectural or geological pattern. Saving a few tiny spots for flickers of red and blue, and for a few lines of the pure, dazzling white of the paper itself, I hunched over the light table wondering how many more layers of gray it would take before I went too far and the whole thing turned to mud. One thing I was finding out was how right Mr. Warnholtz was, that black enriched by other colors always spoke more than the flat color straight out of the can. I leaned over to cut the square shapes of the stencil for which I'd just mixed a purplish blackberry color that reminded me of home, my mother's cobbler, and a bruise I'd once gotten when my horse had stomped on my toe.

Then I heard it, in disbelief: Mr. Warnholtz's motorcycle, buzzing in from a distance and coming to a halt somewhere close. It can't be, I thought, it must be someone else. I had never seen Mr. Warnholtz on campus during a weekend, except when visiting artists came or at a reception for a show opening. Living with his wife on a farm well outside of town, he had a separate, well-protected existence away from us. It can't be, I thought again.

Then came the jangle of keys, one of them turning in the lock of the building's front door, right across from the silk screen studio, and I realized there was no hiding place. This was it. My back to the door as I sat before the light table, I stiffened in preparation for the inevitable tongue-lashing. Mr. Warnholtz's footsteps echoed up and down the hall as he crossed directly to the studio door and proceeded toward me. He's wearing his motorcycle-riding boots and his denim, I thought, the old coot.

But I didn't move, just waited, trying to continue cutting the stencil smoothly, as though nothing could be more ordinary. Maybe he wouldn't notice the prints stacked on the rim of the table above me. But, really, I figured he somehow already knew— that's why he had come.

He stood in silence a moment, then said good morning in his gravelly voice. Because I didn't want to look at his angry face, I continued cutting as I grunted hi in return. I felt his eyes moving like a premonitory tickle across my head and hands, the paper, the X-Acto knife, the can of purplish black ink. He was going to kill me.

Instead, he cleared his throat and shuffled his boots, and so I glanced up at his eyes peering over the rims of his thick glasses, his wild eyebrows like furry, sideways exclamation points. "Do it bigger," he said. Then he took off once more on his motorcycle, leaving me on my own, unbounded.

As I grew up, the official medical word was that I could do anything I wanted to do with my life. Well, except to become an airline pilot, bus driver, or any other kind of employee in control of large equipment or public vehicles. A military career was also likely out of the question. Technically, I suppose most any profession is open to us. I've known of diabetics who were C.P.A.'s, philosophy and biology professors, environmental scientists, doctors, elementary school teachers, and bank executives. The American Diabetes Association is fond of trotting out professional athletes and entertainers like Mary Tyler Moore, our one enduring symbol in the public sphere.

Nonetheless, I found it impossible to remain—or become—a visual artist, and I know that diabetes had a lot to do with that, though certainly it wasn't the only factor. Perhaps if I had gone straight to graduate school, perhaps if I'd had more ambition or patience, perhaps if I'd maintained better control of the disease and had therefore had more energy, perhaps if I'd simply had more talent. My shorthand way of thinking about it, however, is that I had to have health insurance.

I spent several years searching high and low for a career, changing locations and changing jobs, going back to school, volunteering, interviewing, attending career workshops, asking for favors from friends, filling out applications, joining nonprofit artists' groups, schmoozing, trying first to consider wage earning a separate thing and then to channel my visual interests into graphic design. I despised it all and felt miserable, and, though I hated to, I began to give it up, turning eventually to my abilities as a writer, editor, and teacher, whereby it proved somewhat easier to make a living—with benefits.

Inch by inch, choking and squirming through sleepless nights, I gave up the practice of art. Already, before there were any significant complications from the disease, it limited me, boxed me in, made me give up my simple dream of being part of the artsy avant-garde. Looking back, I'm not sure I had the callousness necessary for that lifestyle anyway, but then I just felt trapped. And scared. Admitting to myself that diabetes loomed as a real factor in my life choices opened up a door to all kinds of just-under-the-surface monstrous possibilities. The primary dread for me at that time was, logically, going blind from diabetic retinopathy, a condition wherein tiny blood vessels in the retina rupture, leaking blood into the eye. Already nearsighted, I had worn glasses since fifth grade. But another specter haunted me—that of my elderly biology professor at Carleton, diabetic for many long years and blind as could be, whose wife led him to class and wrote things on the chalkboard for him as he lectured.

Diabetics are four times as likely as others to go blind, and, though I might not be able to imagine what it would mean to develop heart trouble or to be on kidney dialysis, all I had to do to presage blindness was to close my eyes for a while. Then, the shadowy shapes and lurid oozing colors that played across my eyes made the outside world seem orderly and harmless by comparison.

During this period shortly after college, I also experienced my first really sudden low blood sugars, ones where I fell prey to hypoglycemic unawareness, a common condition for long-term diabetics who may have suffered some nerve damage, or just occasional inattention from burnout. When younger, I noticed the classic low blood sugar symptoms when my glucose hit 70, certainly by 60; now it is more often below 50 by the time I stop to check it, frequently below 45. Instead of experiencing the simplest symptoms on the way down, as my blood sugar falls, I shake, get chilled, turn pale, and perspire only on the way back up, once I've treated the low blood sugar. In general there is great variation in low blood sugar reactions—sometimes they are straightforward and taken care of with a glass of juice; sometimes, however, they prove exhausting and I can't recover until I've slept for an hour or two. Usually the latter is the case when the low has sneaked up on me, and frequently I've experienced what's called a "brain reaction," where no symptoms occur until my brain is so devoid of sugar that functions begin shutting down.

One of the first to go is vision. An early one of these episodes happened when I worked as a proofreader for a law firm and took graphic design classes part time at the University of Tennessee. I'd been working eight hours a day at the office, then going to class, doing homework, doing volunteer editorial work for an art magazine, trying to continue with my own printmaking in the basement of my house, and seeing a married man. Clearly, stress had reached a high point in my life, and one day at work, poring over the commas in some lengthy document, I realized that I couldn't make sense of the words. Swarming all over the page, the letters transformed into gnats and zoomed at my face until my eyes seemed covered by insects. When I lifted my head to look around, I noticed huge blank areas in my vision, beige-colored and floating, as well as a closing ring of blackness around the periphery of my sight. I could see almost nothing but this tunnel with clouds passing through.

I know now that these visual disturbances during hypoglycemia are not necessarily related to the retinopathy, glaucoma, and cataracts that plague so many diabetics, but then it made the experience of blindness seem very close and real. How could I plan on a future as a successful artist when I might not be able to see in a few years? My visual sensitivity, perhaps even my choice to study art, suddenly also seemed related to this aspect of my life with diabetes: I had been staring hard, trying to soak up the look of everything in the world, to memorize, to be able to recall the sight of the wind in a stand of silver maples, the Maxfield Parrish blue of the twilight sky, the particular angle at which cats' whiskers flicker when they yawn, my own wavering and dimly pleasant golden oval reflection in a pool of brackish green water. Years later, I would find the same sentiment expressed by Alice Walker in her essay "Beauty: When the Other Dancer Is the Self," about a childhood accident that blinded her in one eye: "I realize I have dashed about the world madly, looking at this, looking at that, storing up images against the fading of the light."

I felt as though giving up art meant a declaration of the coming darkness. Continuing with it, however, seemed impractical at best, a long, selfish, futile struggle. In college, I had garnered praise and attention in the small academic community, winning "distinction" for my senior exhibit and evoking campus-wide discussion about my strange work. Out in the world, no one but me cared whether I ever made a print or sculpture again. Even when I tried to turn to commercial art, I faced the likes of one graphic design instructor who told me that I shouldn't worry, there were plenty of jobs for mediocre graphic artists. Utterly offended, I told her she should look at my record, but I nonetheless knew there was truth in what she said. I couldn't rally much interest in the ideas inherent in the realm of commercial art.

It occurred to me that my fear of blindness had misled me, channeled me into an area of study where I really had little talent. People appreciated my writing and editing skills, no matter in which realm I exercised them—academic, creative, or commercial. I began writing stories and poems as I had in high school and making a living writing ad copy and public relations material. There was a struggle and effort in this work, but it came easier and always held my attention.

My search for satisfying work was not, however, by any means complete. In many ways, I relived, over and over, my experiences in high school, with my doctors, with my parents. Optimistic to begin with, always competent and productive, I would become gradually disillusioned with the irrationality of the workplace, and I couldn't bear to suffer under conditions that made no sense to me. In the ten years after I graduated from college, I held at least that many different jobs in addition to taking classes in a couple of other fields. Somehow, I just never quite fit in.

Though I had always enjoyed writing, I never intended to become an English teacher. Being from a long line of educators—both of my grandmothers, one grandfather, and both of my parents—I knew the pitfalls of teaching as a career. My grandparents and parents had all labored hard for what they believed in, to help others, to make the world a better place, and none of them had been more than moderately rewarded. Like art—and unlike the fields of computers or insurance, where decisions that affect us all are left to the experts who also happen to be making high profits—education invites all kinds of commentary and criticism from a virulent and ill-informed public. As an educator, one gets only intermittent respect and is drawn into constant conflict. Until I was chained eight hours a day to a desk in an office, however, I never fully appreciated the flexibility and variety offered by an educational, especially a college or university, lifestyle.

Working at 13-30 Corporation shortly after I graduated from college, first as an administrative assistant on a project placing sports news posters in bars and bowling alleys and later as a proofreader for all of the company's single-advertiser publications and *Esquire*, I developed the metaphor of erasure for what I felt happened to me when I walked in the door in the morning. Even though 13-30 had a reputation as a cool place to work and jobs there were widely coveted in Knoxville, the dull conventions of each day made me feel as though I were disappearing. I envisioned a silent monster always after me with an eraser; some days it didn't make much progress, but others I would be going home with barely more than my toenails. During the evening and night, my real self would regenerate, but if I had been erased down to my toes that particular day, then I might have to go in to work the next morning still missing my head or my hands. That gave the eraser demon a jump start, and the cycle might go through a horrible phase where I couldn't restore myself and so hardly knew myself, barely felt that I existed.

Later, after moving to Pennsylvania and getting a job as a writer and editor for Penn State University's alumni magazine, I found a boss who allowed me, even encouraged me, to have opinions. But still I chafed at the routines, never-ending, recycling through an invariable two-month process of doing interviews, transcribing, drafting, editing, and proofreading. Everyone I interviewed—the engineer tracing patterns in a wind tunnel, the history professor famous for his compelling lectures about the Nazis, the agriculture dean with photos of pork roasts on his wall—seemed thrilled about his or her work, to carry a faith in its importance that I certainly didn't have in mine. The challenges of my job had faded, it had become easy most of the time, and I found myself secretly writing short stories at my computer during slow times. I had also begun to apply for jobs in other places, feeling an old restlessness that now combined with a despair about running from one thing to the next. It had never been my intention to become a dilettante.

Finally, one August afternoon as I drove home from an interview and job offer in Washington, D.C., as the hills undulated in the heat around my ribbon of road, I realized that this kind of lateral move would make me no happier. A similar salary with big-city expenses would mean a grinding financial struggle, and I would have to prove myself all over again, perhaps with a boss far less amenable than my current one. For a hundred miles or so, the tears coursed down my cheeks and I contemplated Thoreau's notion of quiet desperation. I could get into a car and drive hundreds of miles and still be getting nowhere.

Fortunately, my resolve and stubbornness kicked in, and by the time I reached Pennsylvania 220, turning north from Bedford and shooting along beside a high ridge above a blue-green valley, I had decided the time had come to dig in and build. By the time

I left State College, I vowed, I'd be moving forward, not just away. Here I was, employed by a major university with a tolerant supervisor, and I hadn't taken advantage of it at all.

When I went in to work the next Monday, I asked for a promotion and for permission to adjust my schedule to take some classes. Held up in the glacial bureaucracy, the former would take seven months and would come only a few weeks before I turned in my resignation to become a full-time graduate student, but I enrolled in a class almost immediately. A nonfiction writing workshop with the legendary and ferocious Paul West, this class would, as they say, change the course of my life. Every Thursday afternoon, I left the magazine office and ventured downtown to the conference room where the class was held, as self-conscious of my hose and heels as of my non-degree student status, my stuttering stories. Paul, dressed in soccer shorts and a pink oxford-cloth button-down shirt, held court at the end of the long table and frequently fiddled with the air conditioner protruding from the wall beside him. Arrayed around the table, the motley assortment of graduate students vied for Paul's attention, alternately leaping into the conversation with passionate conviction and leaning back with an affected air of nonchalance. I had no idea what was going on, but Paul's continually fascinating commentary held my attention fast. Though I floundered, I was not bored, and, so, even though I received my share of harsh criticism, I was hooked.

Within a matter of two months, I went from cranking out soured romance stories to crafting a bizarre and tortured experimental piece about the experience of hypoglycemia, and all the credit goes to Paul, who pushed hard, whose spoken vocabulary wheeled like stars in the firmament, who gave me a photocopied page of Proust with the instruction to read it every night before I went to sleep. None of the other students in that first seminar knew what to think when I showed up with this wild piece of writing—it had outdone their critiques based on my status as an unimaginative dullard trying to edge my way into their ranks. At the beginning of class, a fidgety silence fell, and a few ventured mild reprimands for my having broken all the rules they'd said I'd followed too closely before. Paul, however, who has Type 2 diabetes himself, and, even more important, loves any flight of lingual fancy, became at once my friend and champion. " 'Flours,' " he noted about one phrase in the piece, "I've never seen that used in the plural before. Bravo." Breakthrough.

In my transformation from hack to literato, words began to speak a new language to me, a language of discovery and exploration, one in which the scenery lit up at my own thought, in which I could invent colors and shapes and make others see them, too, sometimes. I could take suffering and render it beautiful, or at least bearable. I began, too, to understand the relationship between form and content and, therein, between my self and my words, between my own body and soul: distinct yet inseparable. Lawyers must pass the bar exam, doctors must be licensed, and, in terms of the visual arts, I always waited, hoping to but never really earning the title of artist. Within a few months into my M.F.A. program, however, I knew that I was a writer. I had interesting things to say and, now, tools with which to explore them. My words might falter as much as my body, but between the two I would exist.

At first my intention had been to earn an M.F.A. in nonfiction writing, to bolster my magazine writing career, to make it possible, perhaps, to work for the likes of *Smithsonian* or to at least make up for my bachelor's degree in art, which sometimes held me back when job descriptions listed "bachelor's degree in English or journalism preferred," but a gradual change began to take hold. As a full-time graduate student, I also became a teaching assistant, which in the English department at Penn State means you are given your very own course to teach—no sitting in a professor's undergraduate courses, no grading for someone else, no holding study sessions only; rather, you are given a syllabus and lesson plans, go to a weekly meeting for other new teachers, and run your own classroom immediately.

I took to teaching like a sparrow to air, a duck to water, a pig to mud, a horse to oats. Moving back and forth between life as a student, where, under the best of circumstances, I was pushed and prodded, freed and emboldened, and life as a teacher, where my students might be difficult but where sometimes I could make a light come on, I began to think a lot about power. In all walks of life, some people wield their power in order to squash others like bugs and others use theirs to hold up the world, Atlas-like. Which each of us will be constitutes one of the most fundamental questions any of us answer, and the former type seems to run rampant over the earth.

Though sometimes it seems that generosity can exist only when someone has a surplus of power, it doesn't really matter how much prestige a given individual possesses. I think of the day my mother and I were trying to get ready for her second husband's funeral. Owen had died unexpectedly of a blood clot after heart bypass surgery in a location far from home, and my mother, depleted and bereft, had not been in her own house in more than a month. In my own haste to drive to Virginia Beach from Pennsylvania, I had forgotten to bring extra blood glucose test strips, and since my mother was also short on supplies, we made a trip to a large chain drugstore around the corner from her house.

We still had a three-hour drive ahead of us, as Owen's funeral would be in Alexandria where he had lived most of his adult life.

Equipped with my doctor's phone number for prescription confirmation, I approached the woman at the pharmacy counter. "The doctor will have to call us, not the other way around," she sneered, after I had explained the funeral situation, and so my mom and I went off in search of a pay phone. Done, and a half hour later we returned to the store, filled up a hand-basket with shampoo, panty hose, and toothpaste. Since it was midmorning of a weekday, the store echoed, virtually empty, but when I asked if the woman had readied my prescription, she screwed up her flat lips in her fat face, meandered back behind the counter, and reported that it would be at least another hour.

"But there's no one else here," I said. "Can't you do it now?"

"Prescriptions," she snorted, clacking her long, pink fingernails on the countertop, "are filled in the order in which they come in."

"My mother," I pointed out, "doesn't really want to be late for her husband's funeral. And no one else is waiting. This doesn't make sense."

The bitch just stared, a gleam of vicious pleasure flickering in her eyes. My mother, her eyes filling with tears and her body beginning to collapse under this mindless cruelty, stood passively, the heavy basket of supplies sagging in her grasp. At that moment I recalled the locally owned pharmacy just another mile up the road, more expensive but nicer, and I took the basket from my mother's slack hands, dropped it with a clank to the floor in the middle of the aisle, and led my mother toward the door. "Fuck you," I said over my shoulder.

We were in and out of the other store in ten minutes, the pharmacist as kind in her small way as she could possibly be, volunteering to confirm the prescription status with my doctor later so as not to hold us up and slipping into the bag a package of pocket tissue packs, which my mother would later find indispensable. As we left, she called out afterward, "I'm terribly sorry for your loss. Take care." It was her kindness, and not the other's cruelty, that brought tears to my eyes.

Paybacks, I thought, different paybacks. No doubt that the overweight woman in the Revco had been damaged by parents who cared more about their beer—or their fingernails—than about her, by boys who had taunted her for her chubby cheeks, by overworked teachers who had smacked her palms with rulers, by bosses who told her never to make decisions on her own. No doubt she had a closet full of traumas, an apartment full of dead hopes, a body wracked with its own pains and failings. I could see in my own resentments about the unfairness of the universe, my illness, my lack of love that I could easily grow as mean as her. I didn't want that.

So I chose a path in which the point is handing power, however much or little I may possess, to others—teaching—and where I can share a vision, if necessary without eyesight—writing. Not that academia is pure joy and pleasure—pay and job security are a nightmare, hours are long and lonely, the politics stink like rancid lettuce, and scholars receive little respect in this anti-intellectual nation of ours. When the teaching itself goes badly—and often it does—there is nothing so frustrating and sad. However, when it goes well, that feeling of sharing power, of having my own electricity branch out into arcs of secondary lightning, reverberates like a companionable thunder that I have created myself.

One of my all-time favorite teaching moments came during the first day of November in 1994, my third year of teaching and my fourth time teaching introductory fiction writing. The day had started off warm and oppressively cloudy, but around the time I walked to class wind whipped up through the huge elms lining Penn State's central mall. Rain began to spatter like buckshot, hard and cold, just as I gained the building. In the classroom, the tall windows, opened by earlier inhabitants of the stuffy day, clanked against their frames, and I could hear the trees moaning and creaking outside, the drops of water slapping the leaves and sidewalks. I wiped the moisture from my cheeks, shook out my hair, and laid my lesson plan and books out on the table as usual.

One by one, my students burst in, Matt slinging water from his notebook, Andy dashing across the hall for paper towels to dry his glasses, Jennifer sniffing excitedly at the smell of ozone seeping in through the open windows, Estelle whooping at the relief of reaching shelter from the increasing wind and thunder. They began to settle into the circle of desks around the perimeter of the room, but continued to glance toward the echoes of cars and buses on College Avenue and the shrieks of people getting drenched outside. Each time another student opened the door, they rustled like a flock of restless crows on the verge of flight.

After the last few had straggled in, I tried to lead them around to the day's lesson about how style contributes to theme and meaning and to introduce one of my favorite exercises—how to write a long, hundred-word sentence. By this point in the semester, my rapport with the group was good, and everyone tried valiantly to concentrate, occasionally glancing left or right but mostly looking at their papers. Still, they could not stop giggling, whispering, elbowing, and, after one huge clap of thunder and an increased deluge of rain, Steve's scrawny frame rose from its seat, arms uplifted, hair floating in an electrified nimbus, and he shouted, "I've got to go out in it!" Instantly, he seemed to disappear, leaving only his notebook and the heavy thud of the door behind him to testify to his existence. Then we heard his voice outside, yodeling to the rain gods to bless him and all the world.

Inside, silence.

My students looked at me and I looked at them. We all knew that Steve was a free spirit, even a flake; everyone was aware that he sometimes came to class stoned, and he had been shocked when I'd told him so; because he often staged attention-getting events, he wasn't popular in general, but in this instance he had reached for the brass ring, and everyone was with him. What would happen? A few put their hands over their mouths to stifle their laughter. Others literally sank in their desks, clearly fearful that I would explode in an anger more fierce than any thunderstorm.

I cleared my throat. "Okay," I said. "I give up. There's no use fighting. We will abandon my plan for the day. BUT," I went on, waving my hand in the air as they relaxed and began again to fidget, "you have to shut up right now and write about it."

"Write about what, exactly?" one of my students asked.

"The storm—whatever you're hearing, seeing, feeling, smelling, thinking right now or in the past few minutes. What associations come into your mind? What does it make you think of? Do you hear that bus howling through the wind?"

Instantly, all heads bowed toward paper, hands pushed pens across pages, every mind willingly turned to the task of capturing the moment, of expressing something in words, of learning about their experience through writing about it. What more can a teacher ask for? To sit in a room with twenty other people who have taken what you've given them and made it suddenly their own is stunning indeed.

Ten minutes later, when Steve came reeling back through the door, prepared to interrupt us with his superior experience once again, he found a room full of writers, diligent, absorbed, unstirred by his entrance. "We're writing about it," I told him, and, mouth open, he slipped back into his seat and took up his own pen.

At the end of class I would tell them, "That's how you be a writer." In the meantime, I sat and watched them, moved, basking in the power to give and to find out through language. We seemed like the highest bank of lightning-filled clouds, flashes flickering back and forth between us.

Never mind that I should have begun learning Braille yesterday. Tomorrow will be soon enough.

7

Love Sickness

Tom ignored me. I'd hardly heard from him all summer, but I had hoped for something of a reunion when we returned to college for junior year, as we had been intensely involved the previous spring. Instead, he pretended that I did not exist, that he did not see me studying in the library, that we were virtual strangers passing on the street. At first, disbelief spread through me: this was Tom—Tom who shared my love of cartridge pens but who always seemed to make them leak, who had written me poems with his ink-stained fingers; Tom of the long moonlit walks in the lilac groves; Tom of the funny metallic smell—like the strings of his guitar, played until his fingers, calloused and ridged, stopped and strummed my lips for kisses to alleviate their pain; political Tom, full of moral outrage about apartheid in South Africa, about the plight of the poor, who couldn't bear the thought of anyone being treated unfairly (hah); a Tom of kindness, who had told me not to worry about being transparent, rather that I was apparent, a wonderful quality. Where had he gone? How could this be?

For years and years these questions have recurred in regard to my love life, this continuing disaster of my relationships with men. Over and over, I wonder how someone can change so dramatically, can veer away so suddenly. Even treated cruelly, I cannot change my mind so completely about them. By nature loyal and constant, I discover a stranger in my lover and find myself pushed into a corner with disappointment and mistrust, but only rarely do I cease to love him.

That Tom would not even bother to talk to me about what was going on angers me now, but those were the late seventies, and no one even believed in obligation. Somehow or another, I was supposed to read the handwriting on the wall and get out of the way, move on, accept whatever happened at face value. No one ever took sides in these cases. No protest arose from our many mutual friends at his treatment of me. There were shrugs all around. By the end of the term, Tom would approach me and say that he wanted to be friends, that his anger had subsided and he didn't want things to be awkward between us anymore.

"What on earth have you had to be angry at me about?" I asked, sincerely incredulous as I stood in the hallway of the house he shared with my friends. He had been playing "our" songs in an adjacent room as I visited with Audrey that evening and stopped me as I got ready to go home.

He shook his blond bangs in a certain puppylike way he had and squinted as though looking far into the distance. "The pressure," he said, "the pressure."

Although I had instincts sane enough to be appalled at this

inversion of the situation, I didn't have the nerve to tell him how off base he was. He went on to say that he really didn't want to discuss it in detail, but thought we should get together for breakfast some weekend morning, just to "normalize" things, to reestablish a friendship, to chat. This was as close as Tom ever came to an apology.

As in so many other ways, other situations, I did not know what to do with my grief. No outlet, no ceremony, no ritual existed for me to deal with the loss of my boyfriend, as none existed for my feelings about my disease, my shame over my imperfect body. In fact, these feelings flowed together in a current of paralyzing frustration, and, powerless to change anything, I went through the first days of the school year in a stupor, bewildered, dazed. Too much was happening—Rachel had just informed me that all my housemates were lesbians; one of my friends had been arrested for drug possession; the intensity of my academic life had increased; and my entire social sphere had collapsed.

My own culpability also weighed on my mind. After all, a mere four days after the start of the school year, I'd been back in bed with my old boyfriend Rod, who I had continued to adore in spite of his own impossible nature. Perhaps Tom had sensed this all along, perhaps if I had been purely faithful to him, body and soul . . . perhaps, perhaps, perhaps. Certainly, if I had been prettier . . . I searched for my own errors, I feared my own flaws. But I also knew already from Tom's silences during the summer, from his absence in the first few days back, that he no longer cared, and I badly needed some kind of confirmation, affection, reassurance.

Not that Rod was a great place to get it. No doubt he would give it only to take it away once again, as was his habit. But there on my doorstep one afternoon he appeared, a sight for sore eyes, a distraction, a stable instability. He had bothered to come and find me, and I let him follow me up the dusty stairwell to the second-floor apartment at Bridge Square, carrying a six-pack and bumping me playfully from behind, his hot tongue in and out of my ear. He offered me a beer, and we sat across from each other in a tiny room my housemates and I called the parlor, looking out the wall of windows onto the town square and the little, green Cannon River, the Malt O'Meal factory beyond. Whether we loved each other or not, we certainly excited each other, and our pleasure in each other's presence pulsated between us in our words and gestures. Rod was such a joy to me when he was in this kind of mood—restless, expansive, funny. He told me that he'd tried to live out the summer in a tent in the school's arboretum, but had been caught and ejected, so he'd had to get a job pumping gas in neighboring Faribault. I held his oily, cracked fingers in my hands, turning them to and fro, raising them to my nose for whiffs of his day's activities, and every now and then he'd remove one hand to run it up my arm or to tickle my knee. Then he would set it firmly back into my palm and would smile into my face.

Soon enough, we pulled apart for sips of our beers, and he leapt up in search of music, his stereo long gone for drug and rent money, his longing for sound intense. I followed him into the living room, to the crates of albums, where he had already pulled out Eno's *Taking Tiger Mountain by Strategy*, one of my favorites, to which Rod himself had introduced me. Like pinballs we bounced around the room, touching and avoiding touching, until the seemingly inevitable happened and we wafted back to my cool blue bedroom, the walls hung with Indian prints and two twin mattresses made up on the floor as an oversized and very comfortable bed.

After Rod and I made love, we lay among the tousled covers,

finally relaxed enough to continue our conversation more calmly than before. He wanted to know what classes I was taking, how my parents had responded to my declaring an art major, what art I had seen over the summer and what it had "done" for me. Eerily, however, as though a cold fog seeped through the room, I began to feel guilty. Here I'd been in an outraged fury about Tom, but had been completely willing to hop in the sack with Rod. In fact, I preferred being with Rod, and I always had, but I knew he was a fatal, tragic longing never to be fulfilled. He could never be depended upon for anything. A skirt was irrelevant: Rod slept with anything that moved. Here today, gone today. In one orifice and out the other. I had a whole list of twisted clichés with which to describe him. Tom at least, for a while anyway, had seemed sane and considerate, even temporarily faithful. As I lay there with Rod's arms so casually around me, his fingers stroking, now idly, that patch of skin underneath my arm, his breath against the back of my sweaty neck, a few mercury tears slid down my cheeks into the pillowcase. Seeing my sadness, Rod turned my face to his, traced his finger around the curve of my cheek, and kissed my eyelids before asking me what was going on.

Embarrassed at my audacity and fearing that he would point out my own hypocrisy, I told him about Tom's nastiness.

"That asshole," he said, all sincere concern and outrage. "Do you want me to beat him up for you?"

We laughed and laughed at that idea, both knowing how strange it was for me to garner sympathy about one heartbreaker from another, and then Rod held me while I cried the tears that my other friends had forbidden. I cried, too, at his beautiful acceptance of my own illogic—crying for one while sleeping with another—though of course I didn't tell him about that. His gentleness, his condemnation of Tom's behavior—these were the closest I ever got to an apology from Rod.

At the time, I wasn't even sure either one owed me an apology. In those days our female rhetoric swelled with the idea that we could forge new kinds of decency, a reality in which sexual experimentation might be acknowledged and accepted, where people did not own each other. What we did, instead, was give men permission to abuse us, a reiteration of the form of battery based on the denial of our value as individuals. We became one rotating mass of female flesh to fondle as it passed. The unspoken rule said that we should never complain, for that would mean we were needy and weak, and the last thing we wanted was to be needy and weak.

What made me so vulnerable to this bullshit, I believe now, is that same old primary conflict between my personality and my diabetes, the one desiring to escape the dull limitations of the other. Never able to shut off the practical part of my brain, which kept me taking my shots, I nonetheless wanted my life to somehow reflect strength, independence, wildness. When I discovered that my body could, after all, be the source of pleasure as well as shame and pain and worry, the revelation went awry. Why should anyone put limits on this kind of pleasure, such a rare reward, so unanticipated after years of injections, hospitalizations for hypoglycemic migraines, agonizing menstrual cramps, and the like? For my body to be desired lifted my spirits until I floated above moral and practical boundaries, and Rod could be very direct about his desire for my body. For him, this attached to nothing else, it simply existed for itself; however, for me, the feeling was fleeting enough that I longed to hold on to it through the label of love. I understand now my own tendency to give in so easily to others' desires without ever thinking beforehand of the emotional consequences: otherwise, consequences ruled my life and my physical existence offered me few pleasures. I think now about my tortured body, such a joyful, healthy thing during my childhood, turned suddenly into the overweight, acne-speckled, injected, and often just plain out-of-whack physical entity that it was during my high school and college years. I think it was a wonder I ever got laid at all, and no wonder that I never won love with that body.

Still, long after most of those friends gave up this rhetoric, I live the consequences of it. Within a couple of years of graduation, most of them married; I have not. Then, like Tereza in Kundera's *The Unbearable Lightness of Being*, I thought of myself as retrograde because I really always wanted love and fidelity. My comrades' words echo through my diaries: they thought I was too dependent on others, they told me that having sex with another person didn't change their feelings for me, they said I should grow up, move on, seek change, jump into the kaleidoscope of experience, go with the flow. Even then, I resisted these urgings, and yet somehow I have ended up living them more than those who espoused them. Strange mystery, this, as though all of that adolescent silliness flowed from them into me and pooled permanently in an underground cistern that continues to seep out into my life, effervescent and sweet but poisonous.

When I think of Rod, that fall is my favorite time. By the end of October he would be gone to spend a few months with his older sister in Seattle, probably in some familial attempt to separate him from drugs and alcohol. The next year I would see him again, both in Ames, where he had moved to enroll at Iowa State, and during his visits to Carleton, but he would seem brutally drunk and out of it, charming still but violently self-destructive, and I would finally refuse to sleep with him. A couple of years later, I spoke with him for the last time, when he gave me the news that he was getting married. He had, he said, met a woman who "could really cook—in the kitchen and in the bedroom" and who would go and buy him more beer when he was too drunk to drive. She's fat, he told me, so she'll put up with a lot. What more could he want? All I could think at the time was, Who is this guy? I must've dialed the wrong number. Even if he thought them, the Rod I knew would never say such crude and stupid things. Still, this stranger's words came across the line in his familiar voice to horrify me.

And, yet, how could I be shocked? Rod had already caused me more pain than anyone I'd ever known, in a fashion often so pointedly cruel and irresponsible as to be remarkable even then, in that youthful phase of life, in that selfish era. We had met our freshman year when we lived on the same dorm floor and had partied together all fall while his best friend, Jeff, pursued me with an unrelenting sarcasm and bouts of temper that turned me off right away. As soon as we all returned from the Christmas holidays, I went to bed with Rod, out of a desire for protection from Jeff as much as anything else. Besides, the time had arrived for me to lose my virginity. In fact, I was way past due—already in college and nearly eighteen years old. I was embarrassingly innocent according to the Ann Landers morality test, which we had posted on the lounge wall in order to flaunt our badness. In the process of catching up, which I eagerly did, I seemed for the first time in my life to have a chance at fitting in. It had been hopeless in high school, but now I felt almost in synch.

Lucky for me, Rod was a talented lover, playful, leisurely, and interested in the female body as more than a hole for his penis. So many of my female compatriots complained that sex was a disappointment—"This is it?"—but I enjoyed it from the get-go because Rod had none of those typical young male problems of haste and dominance. We played at long, pointless kisses in the tunnels on our way to dinner; we tied each other to the frames of our little dormitory beds; we tickled each other all over with feathers, gave massages with fragrant sandalwood oil, and lay back on the floor, stoned and naked, our fingers entwined, while the discordance of King Crimson or the ironic beat of Roxy Music danced over us. We would turn toward each other and compare the length of our fingers, our forearms, our shinbones, our full legs, lying on our sides pressed together, staring into each other's black pupils, watching them contract and expand as light and focus changed in tiny increments, our eyelashes brushing each other's cheeks.

Rod also vomited on me on more than one occasion, when he'd come back to our dorm, brimful of vodka or Everclear or whatever was the poison of the evening, always an evening he'd spent with someone else. Someone had to hold his head as he wretched and to make sure he didn't pass out and drown in the puke, and usually that someone was me. Once I spent the entire night curled around him on the men's bathroom floor, my arm cushioning his unconscious head from the cold, hard tiles, keeping him as best I could away from the pinkish gray pools of his puke. Usually, however, when the worst of it had passed away down the toilet, one of the other guys would help me drag him off to bed, where, before I'd leave him to go back to my own room, I'd tuck him in and pass my hand over his forehead like a mother with a sick child.

Of course, he never loved me for this, no more than for my flawed physical attributes, and I suppose that my motivation emerged from wanting to feel that someone might take care of me if ever I got into trouble. No one ever did. The only time I ever came near to passing out drunk while I was in college, I had left a crowded bar and wended my way home through the

Minnesota January by myself. When I lay down on a snowbank, no one else was around, and soon enough I got cold, rose, staggered onward, and put myself to bed.

Rod insisted that the only people he really loved were his little brother and sister, innocent children of elementary school age. What hummed between us he called fondness, and, according to him, it could not be affected by his interactions with others, his visits to a line of other girls. When it came to his interactions with our other acquaintances on the dorm floor, women supposedly my friends, however, the situation often turned ugly. I don't know if Rod ever consciously conceived of himself as being on a mission to sleep with as many people as possible, or if, as it seemed, he just stumbled from one accidental encounter to another. He wasn't even very unusual in this pre-AIDS, post–sexual revolution time, only more extreme.

A few weeks after he and I had first been together, a few weeks during which we had been inseparable as clouds and sky, suddenly, the sun rose fierce and glaring into my romantic haze. My friend Dana had a paper due the next day, and I sat on the floor in her room, proofreading as she clacked away at the typewriter on the desk. One A.M. came and went, the floor quiet on this end-of-the-term night except for a group of bridge players in the lounge, which included Dana's roommate Carol. I didn't like Carol, a worldly-wise daughter of a diplomat who had traveled extensively, lived in Tehran, and put me down as a naïve hick, and I felt certain that Carol didn't like me. However, disliking someone was considered just as retrograde as being possessive, and Carol had always been able to outdo me in faking a benign indifference, even concern. That night, however, she made her hostility completely clear, at least to me. She did so by shining that harsh midnight sunlight on Rod.

About the time the card game broke up in the lounge, Rod

reeled off the elevator, drunk as he often was, and he and Carol came into the room to get high. He patted me on the head, asked in a slur if we wanted to join them, but we continued to work on Dana's paper while on the other side of the room the two of them passed a pipe back and forth and leaned against Carol's mattress, on the floor with no box spring or frame, as was the style. Carol repeatedly whispered in Rod's ear, then cackled her high nasal derisive laugh. His head lolled back on the edge of the mattress, his eyes fluttering open only in brief moments of consciousness, his legs splayed across the rug, Rod grunted once or twice, then passed out.

Carol was having none of that, and she proceeded to unbutton his shirt and massage his chest, heaving herself up to sit on his lap as she did so. Rod's arms rose, slow and stiff, and, his eyes still closed, his mouth hanging open, he ran his hands down her back to her buttocks. A groan escaped his lips, his body lurched slightly from head to toe, and Carol leaned over and began kissing him from lips to naked belly button. Dana and I sat transfixed.

I knew that I could do nothing or Carol would circulate the story of my possessiveness and control over Rod, but, finally, after a few minutes of watching this show, Dana got up, pulled Carol away, and shook Rod by the arm. When he finally started and opened his eyes, she said, in a tone of voice both calm and forceful, "Get yourself to bed. You've passed out." He laughed, wiped his hand across his mouth, and fumbled out of the room.

"That's rape," Dana said to Carol.

Carol just laughed and, on her way out the door, said something about how Rod always wanted it. We both assumed that she followed Rod to his own room, but in a few minutes, almost as soon as Dana had resumed her typing and I my reading (with trembling hands), she returned with another guy in tow, a guy who lived on another floor, but whom Carol hung out with sometimes. They smoked a joint, crawled under the covers on Carol's bed, tossed their clothing onto the floor, and had sex, with much giggling and shrieking, while Dana and I finished her paper not fifteen feet away.

I was sickened by this reality, and right then began looking for other answers to the social questions I faced, but I didn't have much success tearing myself away from this decadence. Rod certainly slept with Carol on other occasions, my roommate Audrey spent the night in his room the last night of the year, even Dana had sex with him the following year, though by then it didn't threaten our friendship because she acknowledged my right to know, the validity of my sense of honesty, my stubborn feelings for him. For a while I prided myself on having Rod's number, on knowing what all the other women didn't know; in a drawing class we shared, I was the only one who knew that he had slept with four of us there, and I could tell immediately when we were assigned to do self-portraits that he and his most recent girl had instead drawn each other. I ceased to pursue him, but rather allowed him to fly into my life whenever he chose, at random, bringing me marijuana, a spectacular dragon bong he had made for me, the latest music he listened to, whatever—and he always brought something. I moved on, spent time with other guys, tried to find a real boyfriend in Tom. Still, Rod retained power and at various intervals convinced me to say stupid things over the air at the student radio station, to stay up all night partying when I had an exam the next day, even to participate in a one-time sexual threesome with him and Jeff, who then briefly resumed his bitter and unwanted attentions toward me.

But in the fall of my junior year, we had a sweet few weeks.

Probably, Rod kept company with me so much because no one else would tolerate him any longer. Most women loved a rebel who was still in school, but a gas station attendant? My guess is that few of his former conquests would have anything to do with him. But, ironically, with little money for alcohol and drugs, Rod in those days often came to me far more coherent than he'd ever been before, and gentled besides. He seemed tired and as grateful for my company as I was for his. It's the closest I've ever come to a sense of what it might be like to settle into the routines of marriage with an intense love that would mellow over time. And yet there was nothing predictable or committed about it— he came whenever he pleased, assuming he could hitch a ride from his place down the road in Faribault; didn't have a phone, so I couldn't call him; and sometimes missed me when I was out with friends or studying. The inevitability of his departure for Seattle gave everything a predetermined feel and kept me from having many foolish hopes.

As it happened, Rod would be leaving the same weekend my parents came to Carleton for their first-ever campus visit, an awkward coincidence if ever there was one. On the day of their expected arrival—via air from Knoxville to Minneapolis, then by rented car to Northfield—Rod showed up around noon as I paced the apartment waiting for them to come. We sat again in the little room overlooking Bridge Square, as we had that first day of the fall we'd seen each other, staring out the windows, making comments about the passersby, reading poetry out loud, he sometimes using an annoying falsetto in order to get me to bristle so that he could kiss my charged lips. We stared out the window some more, the sun beginning to descend into our eyes, wondering why the 'rents had not arrived on time, dallying, picking at the exposed stuffing of the loveseat, smiling wistfully at each other, then laughing, then holding each other close, so tight we could hardly move or breathe, until our desire rose and sent us tumbling across the parlor, entry room, living room, kitchen, and into the bed. Surely, we agreed, this would get them to arrive.

Instead, we had our last time together, intense with anticipation of interruption, but with long spaces of play and simple cuddling, of making tents with our feet under the sheets, of licking the backs of each others' knees, of arguing about the merits of Jackson Pollock's paintings.

"Baby puke," he declared.

"You should know," I taunted. "You've certainly produced enough of that yourself."

As the cool twilight fell, the phone jangled in the living room, and I leapt up to answer it, running naked to the receiver with the low, soft laughter still in my voice as I answered. My father, grumpy from being rerouted and stranded in nasty airports all day, reported that they had finally arrived in Minneapolis and would be in Northfield in an hour or so. To my surprise, Rod had followed me, leisurely, to the phone, and, as I confirmed that I could wait for my parents for dinner, still trying to sound businesslike and alone, he came up close behind me and reached his hand out to smooth my mass of messy hair. Then he put his fingers through to my neck and leaned against me, more still than I had ever known him.

Pathetic as it seems to me today, I had never been so happy.

The next morning, however, I was in a panic. My parents had come and we'd gone to a late dinner, then settled them into their hotel room, and by the time I'd shaken free, it was well past the time that Rod and I had agreed we'd try to meet at a dance on campus. Late, at the dance, I'd searched in vain for the sight of his loose, muscular frame and fuzzy halo of hair. We had hoped to meet up again and spend the night together, to extend our little idyll, but neither one of us had been willing to make a big enough deal of it to be sure it happened. I felt foolish and stricken that I would not see him again. My parents had the whole day planned—breakfast at the Ideal Café, then a trip to the art museum in Minneapolis—so the next morning I left Rod an agonized note and a sheaf of sentimental poems at my door in hope that he would stop by, and went off to play the dutiful daughter.

There, by the door at the Ideal, in the only single-person booth in the place, Rod sat, sipping down the coffee alone. My parents gestured from a booth near the back.

"Too incoherent to come and sit with parents," he said. "Partied too late last night." I examined his pale face, the lavender-gray shadows under his eyes, and doubted he'd even been back to Faribault. He had probably left his belongings in a locker at the bus depot before he'd come to see me the previous afternoon. God only knew where he'd spent the night, as he didn't even appear to have had a shower. "I'll come and say hello to them before I go," he added with a pause, "and bye to you."

Sure enough, in a few minutes he strolled back and gave my parents a polite greeting, and there, with that audience, before going off to pick up the letters I'd left him, he lifted my fingers to his mouth and I lifted his to mine, we each pressed them there, let go, and waved as he backed out of the restaurant. It's as though he's blowing me my kiss and I'm blowing him his, I thought. Weird as ever.

In that moment, knowing that I didn't want it this way, I realized this was what it meant to sleep with a friend, this empty-full feeling, this sense of worthlessness and vague disgust at having revealed myself to someone who remained basically unaffected, who waved a cheerful good-bye to all I had shown him of myself, relieved, unburdened, forgetting as quickly as he passed over the horizon. Binge-purge. In such a short time, I had ridden the smooth, ecstatic back of sex and had had my face pushed into its squishy, rotten underbelly.

During those college years my diabetes haunted me like a ghost that I told no one about, fearful that the rational world would merely make fun of me for believing in it. It was virtually never mentioned by anyone, not even the nurses I saw briefly in the college health service for birth control and sinus and yeast infections. While my family had acknowledged a certain need for special care, once I got away from home I felt free—I could essentially not be a diabetic, not in terms of identity anyway. Usually when diabetic teens go into this kind of denial, they do so rather completely and actually evoke *more* attention to their diabetes from others by making themselves very ill. They deny their own responsibility, shifting it constantly back to others who must help, nag, and monitor them.

I did just the opposite. I myself made others' denial possible by not rebelling past the point where I had to be hospitalized. In other words, my diabetes became my own secret—I behaved fairly responsibly to it, so that others would never see it. My life, my boyfriends, even the general run of my other companions, I often think, might have been very different if I had not tried to live this dual existence.

And yet, I don't know. My doctor seems sometimes to be of the opinion that this has nothing to do with my diabetes, that my personality is in this regard independent of my illness. After all, many people with diabetes marry and have ultra-normal love lives. But how can a condition that affects nearly every tissue and substance in one's body not shape the personality, albeit differently in every individual, in a back and forth or round and round that is much like the dance of lovers themselves? I feel somehow certain that my personality and my disease have mated and produced this difficult offspring, this confused love child.

I have the same kind of relationship with my lovers as I have with my diabetes: I'm uncertain whether my luck and experiences have been fabulous, rendering me in touch with a special reality, wise with richness and variety, or whether I've been just plain old screwed over. I have soared high with heady passion, then fallen into the pits of despair and loneliness; the high and low swings of my emotions evoke in my mind the similarly high and low swings of my blood sugar. Nothing in these two realms ever stabilizes very much. As much anguish as my disease and my lovers have caused me, the disease is one that allows me to live long and fully; my boyfriends have usually been highly sought-after, fascinating men who have provided me with great conversation, even inspiration, if not devotion. Unlike many married women, I have never grown bored. And while I don't think many of them would trade their families for my adventures, I'm not sure I'd trade in my adventures now for a wedding ten years ago.

Still, I expected the carousing to come to a close. I anticipated an eventual mutual, committed relationship. Perhaps I wanted to eat my sugar-free cake and have it too.

But once I make such an assertion I question it. Did I actually ever envision a secure love? Perhaps these years really were marred by a deep sense that no one would ever be able to take me in completely—illness, ugliness, and all. My qualities and behaviors as a lover mystify me, and when I characterize myself one way the opposite seems just as true. Sometimes I've been accused of being too dependent on what others think; other times I've been chastised for my aloofness. "You never let anyone close enough to really know you," one friend observed, and yet over and over I've also been told that my honesty and directness are what scares men away. Recently an administrator in my department asked me to take a job as a research assistant for a particularly demanding professor because, he said, I had a reputation for taking no crap, and he thought I was one of few graduate students who would be able to say no when appropriate; on the other hand, I give my lovers too many chances, I forgive them too often, I allow them to control me with their remoteness. I demand little from them and get even less.

And yet, when I look around me at the behavior of other women, it seems I do an average amount of kowtowing, not really categorically less or more than women more successful in their love relationships. I see women giving up so much of themselves in order to keep peace in their marriages, in their relationships, even in their professions. There seems so much that men don't know about their women, that women tone down for the sake of the male ego and the protection it offers them. Many of my married women friends, for instance, flock to me with discussions about how they don't care for sex, even find it rather repulsive. They would rather cuddle with their children than touch an inch of their husbands' bodies. "Now that we're married," one told me, "there seems like less and less reason to do it." Perhaps, I think, they are telling me these things to make me feel better for not getting much sex myself, to make me feel less an outsider in this coupled universe, but, then, they do not alleviate my alienation in other, more obvious ways. I think, in fact, that my perceived lack of sex (and maybe, therefore, sexuality) makes them feel safe in telling me this; if I *were* coupled they would run the risk of encountering a woman happy with her sex life. Also, their comments end with me, as I have no "other half" who might pass the word on to their husbands.

The fact is that I do like sex, and I've begun to think this has contributed to my remaining single. My mother more than once repeated an old adage to me, which she asserted was still essentially true: Men trade love for sex, whereas women trade sex for love. I have never entered into this equation. I have never withheld sex as a punishment, or as an enticement toward commitment. I have seldom considered it a way to please and keep a man. When I discovered sex, it seemed like such a wonder to find that my body could enjoy and be enjoyed that I shared it freely, never without love, never promiscuously, but without any concept that my body might be a commodity.

Maybe the difference lies, once again, with my disease. My body had seemed worthless to me, certainly not a product that a man would sacrifice his freedom to gain access to. But it goes deeper than this, too, I think. While I have certainly covered up the reality of my body as much as most women—perhaps not wearing as much makeup or dieting as much as some, but surely shaving and deodorizing and hiding my period and slipping away for shots—I've been unable to hide it from myself. For me, with my diabetes, I've had to face up to the crudeness of my physical existence, day in and day out, in order that no one else would know. Many women, I am convinced, manage to hide their bodies from themselves as well as others. They convince themselves that only men are these heavy, unrefined, spitting, farting, shitting, pissing, salivating, tongue-searching, sweating, rubbing, belching, jerking off, puking, ejaculating carcasses. Much as I would like to, I can never forget that I am one of those bodies.

But I also find it impossible to let men forget what this means: that their youth will not last forever. If my men have found the usual blissful oblivion in my vagina, it has always been countered by the knowledge in my eyes and on my tongue, the sweet, whispered premonitions of death that escape me.

∙ ∙ ∙

With Rod and Tom I established a pattern I've never really escaped though it has seen numerous permutations, each one unique. First, there's a wild man, whom no rules can hold and who repents not at his own antisocial tendencies. Sometimes, there are two of these in a row, but they are exhausting, and I always end up sapped and repenting enough for the both of us. Then, there comes a man who seems more normal, but who invariably ends up either completely overwhelmed by me or a psycho in disguise, worse than any honest rebel in the world because he lies compulsively. Whom should I prefer—the guy who tells me that he'll never settle down with me or the one who implies (or lies) that he will but doesn't? Why do these seem to be the only choices I can find to make?

Michael was the only exception to this repeated pattern, and even he partook of many of its characteristics, being flamboyant, brilliant, and unable to pay his bills. Troubled as our relationship was, I am convinced he never would have abandoned me and would probably never have cheated on me. That may not seem terribly impressive, but it's more than I've received in the way of devotion from anyone else. Still, when the time came, I needed to leave him and I don't very often second-guess that choice.

When we met, Michael was married to a woman named Nancy, his undergraduate sweetheart turned into a shy recluse of a lawyer. He and I worked together in the tight, tension-filled typesetting department of a national magazine publisher. Often, we worked overtime, reading aloud to each other the various drafts of the material that would eventually become *Esquire, Moviegoer, New Parent Advisor, Nutshell, Destinations*. Often, with groups of other co-workers, we drank together in the Union Café in the ground floor of our office building, blowing off steam from our pressured work days. Often friends from other sources would join the group, but never Nancy. When she came to pick him up, she would sit in the car on the other side of the long windows, staring at the steering wheel, until Michael would leave his half-full beer glass and shuffle out, head down. A gossipy crowd, we all speculated about their marriage, insulted that she seemed to feel too good to join us, too dismissive of Michael's friends to bother to meet us. Even when one of Mike's old college friends—David or Toby or Iris or Fort—would join us, Nancy would not come in. We all noted, without saying it, that she was obese and seemed extremely depressed, and, despite the fact that Mike often carried a few extra pounds on his large frame, she seemed an odd match for his garrulous charm and bright good looks. "In college," David informed us with a sigh, "she was stunning. I don't know what's happened."

After a year of flirtatious friendship, during which I had had only a sleazy one-night stand and virtually no dates, Michael and I began a secret affair. I want to say in my own defense that the idea certainly did not originate with me, but I followed easily where Michael led. I put up virtually no resistance. It had never occurred to me to be interested in him sexually—after all, he was married, and I was a feminist who wouldn't tread on another woman's territory—but I also hungered for male attention, so rare and stingy in those years. One night after a party, Michael confessed in a deluge that his marriage to Nancy was a failure, virtually over, etc., that he had done everything he could for her, begged her to see a therapist, waited patiently, held her hand, but somehow she was lost, changed, deadened by the emotional stress of law school, her sudden lack of stellar success, their mutual grinding poverty in spite of their education, blah, blah, he had watched me for months, could hardly concentrate on the punctuation when I read him a manuscript on breast-feeding, thrilled when I mentioned the softness of my new corduroys, admired my ability to stand up to our demagogic boss . . . that he loved me.

Surprisingly enough, there is no doubt in my mind that he did.

In the beginning, I told Mike that our affair would be brief, a respite for both of us, a flash in the sky, and that then I would leave Knoxville, as I planned to do anyhow, and go off into the world. Three things influenced these attitudes that placed relationships for me in the grip—and release—of constant change: the confused social values of my friends at Carleton; my parents' own less-than-happy marriage; and the prevailing understanding that diabetic women could not safely have children and were, therefore, not good marriage material. In fact, the care guide of the American Diabetes Association, the ominous, navy blue-covered *Diabetes for Diabetics*, stated that although it was possible for a diabetic girl to marry, her father should be sure to sit down with any serious suitors and explain that pregnancy would be at best difficult, at worst tragic or impossible (fetuses often died in the womb in the last trimester), and that she would always be a financial burden. Of course, by the time I reached childbearing age, prospects for successful diabetic pregnancy had improved considerably, but it never had become a part of my self-concept. With Michael, I began to realize the extent to which I had assumed that none of my relationships could develop into anything committed. With him, that pained longing I had momentarily felt at Rod's departure became a regular, if not consistent, part of my psyche. He gave me the only confidence I'd ever had in my own desirability and worth, in the idea that I might be an addend in the balance sheet of life, not a loss. Soon I began to think of us staying together, maybe even forever.

For the most stable love relationship of my life, my five years with Mike were nonetheless a wild roller-coaster ride of conflict, uncertainty, and fervor. His declarations of love and devotion, the chicory and thistle bouquets from the roadside, the elaborately painted boxes with origami-folded meditations, his nicknames for me—all rose and then fell when he would leave me waiting for hours beside the Dumpster in his apartment building parking lot, or when he would litter my driveway with untold cigarette butts because he was angry I wouldn't let him smoke inside, or when he would spend all the money I'd loaned him on new books and beer instead of paying his rent with it.

It took him six months to move out of his wife's apartment, and when she staked out his new place one night and found out he was spending the night elsewhere (with a woman, surprise, surprise), he moved back in with her "to give it a final, fair chance." Although I had never suggested he leave her, I grieved, guilt-stricken and crazy with fear that this had been just another sleazy affair. In a few weeks, however, he moved back out and finally filed for divorce.

Michael agonized all that summer, waiting for the decree to come through, as though he himself were now a man undergoing nightly torture, rather than experiencing the release of telling the truth, coming clean, and being free to pursue his new life with me. Drawn and haggard, his face sank into dark gullies, his eyes rimmed constantly with red and black, their whites yellowing from the ever-increasing chain-smoking. When summer turned into fall, then winter, and Mike still seemed haunted, I feared that he still wanted to be with her, though he assured me this was not the case. He told me that I didn't know what it meant to break this kind of commitment, and indeed I didn't. What sharpened that into this blade of irreparable guilt, however, I would only learn some years later.

At the time, I watched Michael waffle about career choices,

ignore the engineering courses he'd been taking, take to drinking all night with his fellow restaurant workers, and treat me with a strange admixture of adoration and contempt. While he spent hundreds of hours in my mother's garage, using only the most primitive tools and starting with the crudest lumber, building me two monolithic bookcases with notched, adjustable shelves and surfaces as smooth as chocolate mousse, he also drove me crazy with worry by disappearing for hours, even whole days at a time. On Valentine's Day, he said nothing, merely thanking me for my gift and dissembling about being broke—here we were, I thought, finally in a situation where we could indulge our most romantic notions, and he did nothing—but when darkness fell a pebble hit my second-story window and I looked out upon a kiddie pool–sized, snow-rimmed heart, flames leaping from its center into the blue February air. I did not notice the slight taint of lighter fluid wafting away into the cloudy night.

Mike didn't mind my diabetes. In fact, he waxed poetic about the sweet-salty taste of my skin and woke in the night whenever my blood sugar slipped below the safety zone. Coincidentally (or perhaps not), during this time, my need for care increased, and Michael, when he was there, gladly provided it. I suffered several sudden migraine headaches, accompanied by vomiting and hypoglycemia, and Michael grew adept at whisking me to the emergency room for a shot of Demerol and Phenergan and then bundling me into bed and bringing chipped ice and Sprite until I could recover. I liked the feeling of having someone to rely on in an extreme situation, but it also became clear that Michael often created the crises to begin with. I carried a heavy burden of financial responsibility for the both of us and was always in charge except when my blood sugar crashed; he was incapable of keeping regular hours for meals or anything else and would often bring me treats—sweet for the already sweet, he would say. By the time we moved to Pennsylvania for him to go to graduate school, I held down three jobs to support us. He, on the other hand, roamed the local golf course until 4 A.M. discussing Derrida, leaving me all alone within the cold stone walls of unpaid bills. On the other side of the closed windows, the velvet evening sky opened its arms to the contents of my imagination.

Predictably, I fell in love with someone else.

I'm convinced that your pheromones change when more than one person is in love with you. During the time when I was sorting out my choice between Michael and Panos, all kinds of men paid attention to me, in a way that I had never before experienced. One man I met at the gym brought a dozen roses to my office. A powerful New York editor invited me to come to the city so that he could escort me to the Isamu Noguchi museum. A Washington attorney and member of the board of trustees of the university where I worked pursued me relentlessly, sharing his 50-yard-line football tickets and trying to press kisses on me whenever he could. The men in my office, men I had worked placidly with for more than a year, suddenly began a campaign of suggestive remarks; a married one soon asked me, point blank, to have an affair with him. All of this display nauseated me slightly, but the heady feeling of desirability also slipped in under my sternum and grasped the wall of my heart as fast as any pacemaker. I've since grown sarcastic about this lemming phenomenon, this bandwagon mentality, but I still crave the power of that moment.

Perhaps, in all fairness, what compelled all these men was simply the way in which Panos lit me up. Panos had a gaze like a magnifying glass—when he turned it on you, you knew you were observed, and your internal organs began first to melt, then to burn. All I wanted, once his eyes had focused on me, was to be grilled to perfection, to be bitten by those white, white teeth, to have those molars release my warm juices into his mouth, and to slide down his throat into the caverns of his body. At the time I never gave a thought to how I would come out on the other end or to the overwhelming sensation of being flushed away without a further glance. No, then I must have jiggled with the promise of a fresh, fat-marbled steak under its plastic wrap, I must have sparkled like gin flowing over ice, shocked the glans as if I were frigid water in a glaring turquoise pool, glowed like the summer Saturday sunburn or the hot charcoal fire, ready to cook. Ready.

Panos accomplished this for me by one simple fact—he did not seem to be repelled by the reality of bodies, their inescapable unfolding end, their simultaneous all and not-all status. Fastidious in his own habits, perhaps he simply had never been repulsed by his own physical being, but I thought, and still think, that it was otherwise. His mother had died of cancer, and though I also believe he exaggerated his own role in caring for her, he nonetheless certainly knew the smell of rot on the breath of someone he adored. The tumor in his own arm, its sunken patch laced with stitch scars a testament to his own bone-removing surgery, had bound him to his mother in a way that added to the intimacy of her body having given birth to his: they shared a disease and all the secret knowledge that implies, and, in spite of her hideous, drawn-out death, he always referred to her as the flower in the family cesspool. Body was reality, the boundary, but in spite of Panos's protests that we were composed of "only synapses, no soul," he acted as though he also knew the limits of the limit, that the body could not explain itself or its transmutations.

One day after I had been living with him a few weeks, I

arrived back at his apartment after work to find him sitting at his immense heirloom desk poring over a packet of materials from the American Diabetes Association for which he had written off himself without my knowledge or prompting. As I stood, suddenly shy—scrutinized and flattered—in the doorway, he peered up over his wire-rimmed glasses and scrunched his nose. "I just wanted to know," he said. "Now I do."

I felt physically at ease perhaps for the first time in my life. When I disappeared into the bathroom to test my blood sugar, Panos would follow me to the door to find out the result, to stand chatting about his day, to kiss my belly once I'd taken my shot. If we were involved in one of our many heated discussions when he needed to piss, I'd simply go with him, and he would sit to do his business just so he could pull me to his lap there, too. I sat on the edge of the tub and shampooed his hair as he luxuriated in the bath; he rubbed my back when I had PMS; we played at sex off and on for hours, weaving it into the movies we watched, the books we read, the meals we ate, the phone conversations we had. Mostly, however, Panos comforted me by understanding my disease, by always knowing what to do, by getting up with me at night when my blood sugar was low, or by bringing me a glass of orange juice himself so that I wouldn't have to get out from under the covers, and by doing it all as though it was effortless, even fun, even a part of knowing me. The relief of not having to continually explain myself, of having my diabetes be a normal thing we shared, instead of an interruption I'd have to make over and over, lightened me, and I rose skyward over a widening horizon.

This, I realized some years later, must be how healthy people feel most of the time, moving through a crowd like sunlight, touching another's hand with no thought at all, taking the air for granted. With my body's problems so confronted, I felt suddenly less limited by them than ever before, but unfortunately the confidence I got from Panos was only on loan. I wish I had stolen some to keep for myself, but perhaps that is impossible for those of us who are other; the fact is that we simply *are* different, alienated, outside of the standard milieu, unless accompanied by at least one who shares our predicament. Sometimes I bask in a current of warmth, a delight in the memory of that experience, feeling luckier than most, feeling almost blessed, for having known that sensation of saturated love, though it nearly killed me to lose it. Once having known it, returning to days without it was—and continues to be—brick-wall hard. In spite of continuing on, determined to hold up the blue, blue sky, to keep walking until I found a greener valley over that horizon, I still return to that pool in my memory, more often than I like to admit.

Panos infected me with a different gift, too, however, and that was my first STD. In the guise of a harmless, easily cured case of trichomoniasis, he let me know that our disagreements over the nature of relationships, over the role of fidelity and the importance of honesty, comprised more than mere abstractions. His understanding of the body had been acquired, after all, under the tutelage of the whores of Athens, beginning when his grandmother caught him masturbating at the age of eleven. His skin had touched the skin of hundreds of women—virginal daughters of the Greek aristocracy, raunchy children of the United States diplomatic corps, fat British tourists visiting the island of Mykonos, half-starved ebony prostitutes newly in from the plains of Africa, two-bit models and dominatrices with black leather thongs who thronged his investment-banker brother's parties in New York. Our intimacy at times permeated me so thoroughly that I forgot such things, forgot that there existed this entirely other realm where I was neither welcome nor comfortable.

We had already parted ways when my diagnosis came through. We had, after all, virtually nothing in common but this confrontation with mortality and a kind of resultant emotional and physical concordance that had rendered our sex life stellar but our conversations hellish. "You say potAYto, I say potAHto. . ." We fought all the time, about the trivial and the significant, about Dukakis versus Bush (some ancient Greek family plot had turned him against the Massachusetts Democrat); about how much I should eat (always more, according to him); about whether to buy toilet paper from recycled material (absurd tree-hugging, he thought). He insisted that I not come home from work before six o'clock because I would interrupt his own study routine. When his ex-wife enrolled in one of his classes, he strutted and preened that she would do anything to get close to him, and only when I pointed out that one of his numerous departmental enemies might find out and report his use of the classroom for his personal melodrama, or that another student might find out and claim he favored her unfairly, or that she herself might refuse to do her work in expectation of an easy A—only then did he make her drop the course. If I wanted to go for a walk on a beautiful fall afternoon, he would refuse to accompany me, claiming to hate fresh air.

Once, however, I convinced him to go kite-flying under a brilliant April sky, and we laughed and rolled in the grass and watched the multicolored panes of cellophane soar upward in the wind, his eyes reflecting a rainbow of brightness, the clouds gone. In every instance in which I managed to get Panos to let the sun in, he became plainly happy and as sentimental as a child: he nicknamed the groundhog that circled the backdoor Spike; without any fuss he allowed my cats to drape themselves across his sofa's silk upholstery and to curl up inside his mother's Ming bowl; he polished every leaf of the dracaena I gave him. But when he lifted his head in self-consciousness all of this embarrassed him. It was too wholesome. It was as though he feared being caught by the jaded pseudo-sophisticates that inhabited his life in New York and Athens, his investment-banker brother especially. In that world, simple pleasures did not exist. What they considered fun was picking up a runaway teenage girl and passing her around from man to man for a few weeks until they all tired of her. Panos could hardly force the two incommensurate definitions to make sense together.

To his credit, Panos never wanted the sharing of universes to go in the other direction. When I tried to bridge the chasm by dressing up in a masochistic bustier, he insulted me by rushing from the room, a horrified, "That isn't you. You don't need that," sputtering from his lips. I thought then that this was all still a game, that his exclusion of me was unfair. Such is innocence. I didn't realize that it was a game that was so difficult for its players to leave, that its rigid rules soon took control over its participants' breathing. Panos, I am convinced, knew this and left me behind because he could not hide it sufficiently from me.

But in many ways it was already too late. He had come home from a trip to Greece with his brother and had left on me the physical mark of the filthy body, a sexually transmitted disease, the original disease-as-wages-of-sin. In many ways, he was just another asshole. My next two lovers would likewise give me STDs, in an amazing chain of events related to the susceptibility of diabetics to infections of all sorts, to slow healing, to delicate and easily permeated skin. No one—no book, no brochure, no medical personnel—had ever indicated to me that my risks in this regard were any greater than the general population's, probably because no studies have ever been done of this matter.

Diabetics are expected to be saintly in terms of our eating and drinking habits, so of course the same is true for our sexual habits. Hardly anyone ever discusses our sex lives: because so many diabetic men become impotent, perhaps it is assumed that we just don't have such a thing or that we have only the chaste, puritanical, missionary-position version.

Only after I'd been given the gifts of both venereal warts and herpes did my gynecologist suggest that my diabetes might have played a role in my contracting these diseases with the minimal, protected contact I'd had. The warts had blossomed into a rampant case within two months of their first appearance after I'd been with a man who supposedly had been treated and "approved" for sexual activity. They spread so quickly across my cervix that within three months I underwent outpatient laser surgery for their removal. The healing, as is typical with diabetes, took a long time.

Already, I was seeing someone new, and Bill, desperately horny, told me that it had been a long time for him. After my doctor "approved" me as all healed and ready for action, I got herpes from the new guy: in our fourth instance of intercourse, not one of them without a condom. I had sworn that I would never be a sucker again, but there I was in the doctor's office once more, this time with severe pain and a fever of 102 degrees.

"I used to have trouble with that myself, back in medical school," the substitute doctor told me, my regular one being out of town. "Don't worry much about it." I lay on the table, my legs splayed open to this stranger, my mind raging. He did not prescribe the only medication, in that only moment—the first outbreak— that might have permanently reduced my future attacks. He did not care about my sense that, once again, I'd been lied to and betrayed. He did not understand my concerns with having both diabetes and herpes, two drains on my energy, two stress-aggravated problems, two painful and shameful conditions.

Later, my regular gynecologist told me that my skin, because of the previous laser surgery, had probably been thin, more easily permeated by the virus. "Your immune system, with the diabetes," she continued, "may also be weaker than most and couldn't fight off even the tiniest exposure." Why, I wondered, had she told me it was okay for me to go ahead with sexual activity? Why had no one ever told me that my diabetes might render me more vulnerable to these things?

"Even if your boyfriend only had a rash on his thigh, the herpes could have been transmitted to you, with the moist, sugary environment your body provides," the doctor explained further. She paused, almost as if uncertain. "I'm sorry this happened. The things I see," she said, "sometimes make me wonder about men."

But I was forced to wonder whether I had been betrayed by these men or by my own body. Having drinks with a bunch of casual acquaintances one afternoon, I overheard one of them gossiping about a notoriously hot woman in my department. Large-breasted and cow-eyed, she drew admiring comments from the neophyte, but the more seasoned fellow said to him, "Well, I don't think you'd really want to sleep with her, no matter how good-looking she is. She's a slut, and God knows what you might catch." Bitter, my only thought was, No, gadabout that she is, I bet she's clean as a whistle. I knew there was no straight line between bad behavior and retribution, but still somehow I felt that I must deserve all this punishment my body was receiving. That my body started out more vulnerable than most seemed like part of this retributive fate.

As an objectified product on the market of love and marriage, I am no great buy in terms of the main criteria that seem to apply.

Attractive enough but not beautiful; mouthy and bossy but desiring tenderness; no good for childbearing and unwilling to soften my sharp intelligence, I've also been labeled by my friends as too picky for my own good, whatever that's supposed to mean. Unable to bring myself to settle for the kind of desperate men who occasionally want to marry me after two dates and unwilling to accept that the lovers I see as fabulous won't ever tweak themselves just a bit for me, I remain essentially alone, moving through disappointments like a second-rate horse at the race track. After each event, I stand lathered, my legs trembling weakly, nostrils wide from oxygen deprivation and panic, my heart strained, wondering if, once again, I have overestimated my own worth.

All of this, you may say, is my own fault. A hundred truisms come to mind: I've made my own bed, and now I have to lie in it. I might catch more flies with honey than with vinegar. What goes around comes around. My choices have often been terrible, and I have been motivated by fear, vanity, and desperation, all characteristics not particular to those of us with diabetes. And yet I insist that my love story would have had a different plot without it. My sense of myself as an alien, as I've said, contributed to my tolerance for those on the fringe of antisocial sexuality. Soon enough, I would learn the hardest of lessons about throwing out the baby with the muddy bath water. Soon enough, I would be wishing for something not traditional exactly, but solid and decent. Soon enough, I would be sickened by imitation love, the toxic food coloring of insincere romance.

Panos had given me a taste of something I'd never before been sure even interested me—an overwhelmingly satisfying monogamy. For so many of my rebellious college compatriots, a first experience of this sort led to marriage and stability. For me, it became an unful-filled longing, a Holy Grail, something I needed to prove that I was worthy of. Nothing—not all of my adventuring, not the lustful looks of countless losers, not the heady role of hellion—could come close to the fullness and focus I'd felt with Panos, whether he'd been a Greek god or just a goddamn Greek, to quote a joke that someone told me after he and I broke up. His flaws—the short, stocky stature caused by too much ouzo as a teenager, his hair thin-ning along the edges of his brown forehead, the slight gap between his two front teeth, even his immoral posturing—didn't dampen my dedication to him. No matter that Michael was a better human being; justice, I had learned, fled at love's appearance.

Still, the pleasure of the certainty of the feelings Panos evoked hummed inside me, as simple and direct as the sensation of lying flat on my stomach baking in the summer sun on a slab of granite in a Smoky Mountains stream—buzzing, solid, eternal. I sud-denly wanted to be married, to prove that such a feeling could last even through a winter when the creek filled with ice. Such notions led me as far down into the chilly undertow as I ever hope to go: to a guy named Bill.

After my failure to hold on to Panos, I set about changing my ways, dating several men at once, on a casual, nonsexual basis that I hoped would lead to my getting to know them a bit better, to me finding someone who would be marriage material. In addi-tion, I selected several who all seemed to be rather average, not the wild men I'd pursued in the past, just as parents, friends, and therapist advised. For a brief time, one of these relationships, with a computer programmer from my office, developed further, but both of us were really afraid to make any adjustments for the other. He refused to quit having lunch every day with a flirtatious wench from his department, and I had no interest in learning to scuba dive, his consuming hobby at the time. Quiet, shy, sweet, and relatively unsophisticated, he had no means of coping with the aftereffects of Panos, and when he told me that I stressed him out so badly that he was having to stop and throw up on his way to work nearly every day, I told him I was sorry and went back to dating around.

Soon enough I met Bill. The accumulated failures of my love life already flew around me like rabid bats in the night sky, and my own sense of the world seemed about as trustworthy as a B-grade horror movie. Vague swooping shapes, barely visible in the murk, drew closer around me in a tightening circle of threat and dread. I would become my grandmother, who married and had a child, then divorced and spent the rest of her life alone, literally untouched, as though surrounded by the frantic destructive protection of a swarming cloud of rat-faced winged black creatures. By this time I wanted desperately to succeed.

How do I describe what happened with Bill over the next two years? The words that I love so much, in which I invest all of my hopes and expectations, those words that are the main web of connection and understanding in the world, will lack something here. Perhaps I am struck so wordless when I think of Bill because he was such a consummate liar. His words twisted in the air of their own accord, spinning in a million different directions, blinding their recipients by the sheer glare, like a headlight beam fracturing against snow crystals on a windy night road drifted with snow. I kept on driving into it, afraid of freezing to death in a snowbank, but every now and then I got a glimpse of one of those furry black bats against the livid whiteness of his lies.

He lied about everything, even about what the date of his birthday was, so that he might celebrate it with different girlfriends, so that he could make me believe that he was so lonely he sat at home alone on his birthday waiting for my call.

At first Bill had seemed incredibly dependable, showing up on time, calling from the lab to let me know when he'd be done with work, inviting me to sit around and have a few beers watching baseball on TV with his friends and co-workers. To me it all seemed ultranormal, and what I worried about was boredom, that Bill wouldn't be able to hold my interest, to build fires in my mind that would turn into the glowing embers of fascination. I didn't pay attention to the few signs that something might be amiss. One evening early on, for instance, as we sat in Bill's apartment after he had cooked dinner for me, a woman opened the door, stepped into the living room, then wheeled around and fled in obvious shock.

"Jean." Bill leapt to his feet and launched toward the door, calling into the already empty stairwell, a look on his face as blank as a piece of paper on the first day of school.

Immediately, he returned to my side and lifted my fingers to his cheek. "Poor Jean," he said. "She's been a really good friend and has always wanted more than friendship, but I've never been interested in that with her." He paused and looked soberly into my mistrustful eyes. "If you want, you can ask John and Laurie— they're friends with her, too, and know all about it. Just the other day Laurie told me that Jean's really upset that I'm finally seeing someone I really want to be with." He squeezed my fingers and smilingly leaned over to kiss me. Later both Laurie and Jean would confirm that the latter had been sleeping with Bill for more than a year, and more than one other woman would tell me that Bill had told this same story about me.

For nine months I didn't suspect a thing, but then Bill moved to Seattle to take a position as assistant professor. We talked about splitting up, but more often we talked about a temporary separation—until my studies would reach a point where I no longer needed to be on campus and could join him on the West Coast. Cuddled close nights after lovemaking, Bill would whisper into my ear that he wanted to marry me. The following spring he would tell a couples therapist that I'd been pressuring him for marriage and that he just didn't feel ready.

Quite the contrary was true. I had been trying to break up with Bill since a horrendous Christmas visit, but did not seem able to step away, and therein is the greatest mystery of all. He alternately pled and accused, and I accepted blame and criticism as though they were hors d'oeuvres passed around on a tray at a cocktail party, as though they were raindrops falling inevitably from the sky onto my upturned face.

When he backed my car into a post, he said it was my fault because my computer boxes blocked the window.

When he undressed a waitress with his eyes, he noted that I hadn't been paying enough attention to him, that I just didn't understand men, and that I should watch my figure.

When his friends were rude to me, he told me to be more easy-going, to have another drink, to forget about it because they were just jealous and possessive about him. God knows, they must have been aware that I wouldn't be around long.

When he was impotent, he blamed me because my breasts weren't "as big as Julie's." Of course, Jean, a busty woman herself, reported to me that to her Bill had blamed his impotence on the fact that her hair wasn't blond, or some such.

When I had driven three thousand miles with my two howling cats in the car to spend the summer with him, and had found— the very day after my arrival—a sexually explicit note from one of his other lovers, a naïve young woman from Spain who was in the process of arranging to come on a government grant to work in Bill's lab, he blamed the stress of his job, he blamed her for throwing herself at him, and he blamed me for not being there for him. When, after hours of screaming and yelling and crying at the discovery of yet another lie about a woman, Bill essentially raped me, holding my arms while the tears slid down my temples and I squirmed and whimpered a repeated "no," he claimed that he was trying to make up for all that had happened, that I wanted it as badly as he did. "No," I said, "I wanted you to love me, not fuck me. I was just too tired to fight anymore." Later that night I hovered over an open drawer of kitchen knives, shaking with rage. I wanted to kill him. Instead, I locked myself in the bathroom and sobbed under the shower until the hot water ran out. I had two more months to live with him.

Toward the end, after I had called most of the women in his Rolodex and knew what there was to know, Bill wept and begged me not to abandon him. As a teenager, he had been seduced by a friend of his parents and, he said, this had screwed him up. It would take someone who knew, someone as relentless in her pursuit of the ugly truth as I had been, to help him straighten out. But he lied about that, too, calling me on the phone constantly while renewing his affair with a woman working in his department and telling friends that I was harassing him. They never knew that between the end of the August that I left Seattle and the weekend of Thanksgiving—when I told him I never wanted to hear from him again—Bill called me more than fifty times, pleading with me to give him another chance, the most impossible notion I had ever heard.

Why Bill seemed to get his jollies by torturing me and several other women at a time may be a fascinating psychological question, but the one that haunts me is why I so willingly endured this torment for so long. Why did I give him so many chances? Why did I try so hard to believe what he said, following an ever unwinding skein of yarn into knot after knot? Why, even after I knew the gist of the bald and sordid truth, did I continue to feel that I should help him instead of telling him to go to hell? A child of moderate privilege, never abused, never abandoned, I shocked and astounded myself by being in this tawdry, trashy, low-self-esteem kind of position. It just wasn't supposed to happen this way. Could this really be my life?

Somewhere in all of this lurked the fear, the underground belief that we get what we deserve. Intellectually, I had known better for years, had been pushing away the idea at least since I'd left Michael, but I still wanted to *prove* that it wasn't so, that I hadn't done anything to bring this nasty person into my days and nights, that even Bill didn't deserve the repressive mother, her early death, or the sick seduction of the older woman, who created for him a permanent adolescent hard-on associated with secrecy. I wanted the forgiveness of flaws to repair them, to at least buffer their effects. How could I reject someone who was sick, when I didn't want others to reject me because of my illness? Didn't I want someone who could look past my hypoglycemic mood swings, my injection-bruised belly, my strange habits?

But I could never forgive Bill. His humiliation of me was too calculated, too complete, too persistent and unrepentant; the discrepancy between how we treated each other too huge. While I had been packaging up the most beautiful eastern fall leaves I could find to send him in response to his whining about "no autumn" in the Pacific Northwest, he'd been winging his way to a secret rendezvous with Jane in Illinois and taking Claudia dancing. While I'd been turning the silky-lipped Sean away in State College, he'd been having a friend fix him up with a one-night stand at a wedding in Annapolis because, as he told the friend, he'd "been alone so long." While I'd been driving all over Seattle to find him decent bagels, he'd been laying the ground-work for his next conquest, flirting with a graduate student employed in his lab. He lied to me and about me, he told me I was ugly, he made me seem stupid. He took years off my life.

And so, I wish him only nonexistence. I wish he had never been born, but that having already happened, I wish he would die. And as long as he's walking around on this earth, I wish him only suffering.

It changes a person to wish someone harm, and I am the first to admit that I have never fully recovered from this experience. In order not to spread the damage, to absorb it all myself rather than passing it on the way Bill continues to do, I have closed myself off from others, and I have not had a subsequent boyfriend that I didn't regret my involvement with. I have dated mostly the walking wounded, men so low that they've been either so desper-ate to have a relationship of some sort that they can't even bother to get to know me before trying to take over my life, or so selfish and superficial that they see me only as some kind of tem-porary accessory, like a fashionable computer to be replaced by the next model on the market. I am so harmed that only those who want to take advantage of me find me compelling anymore, and I can only envision myself with someone so unworthy that I can't imagine anyone else putting up with him.

Some months after I broke up with Bill, my doctor seemed to have a new opinion about the relationship of all this to my ill-ness. When he and I discussed the possibility of antidepressant medication, I told him about how Bill had blamed his impotence on the size of my breasts. Like a horse suddenly baring his teeth, Dr. Ulbrecht threw back his head and unleashed more than a whinny of laughter. "You can't possibly take this seriously," he said, regaining his somber composure. "That's as ridiculous as anything I've ever heard. Why would you even speak to a guy after that?"

Sitting there in his office, constantly aware of the contrast between the efficient, cheerful voices of the nurses in the hall and the shrunken, barely discernible sounds of their patients, I could hardly concentrate on Dr. Ulbrecht's words. I knew he was right, but something about his—and the nurses'—easy certainty floated beyond my grasp. I just couldn't apply it to myself. I remembered how my old, old friend Dana had expressed her shock when I'd filled her in on Bill. "Lisa!" she gasped. "What were you thinking? That kind of bullshit is completely unacceptable. If you ever find yourself in that kind of situation again, just call me, and I'll tell you in no uncertain terms to get the hell out." Everyone seemed to know this, everyone but me. Perhaps for the first time, I felt like a victim, like a sick person. I had only been pretending to be one of them—normal, sane, healthy.

"This kind of thing is common among the chronically ill," Dr. Ulbrecht said matter-of-factly. "You may feel that you don't deserve any better, that your diabetes means you have to put up with this." Before he even said the words I quaked with the ever-stronger realization that this might never have happened to me, that I might never have allowed someone to treat me this way, if I had not had diabetes. I thought about all those old patients I had seen so many years earlier at Dr. Gilbertson's—beaten down by years of sickness, psyche following body like a whipped dog.

What could I do but hate my disease even more than before?

So Bill formed this great divide, a Grand Canyon in my life, between optimism and pessimism, where I now dwell. Before, I could pretend that nothing was seriously wrong with me; afterward, the jig up, I came face-to-face with my ailing self.

For a while, I still tried to preserve the notion that I could heal the damage in my life, that it was not something permanent and incurable. I went to Michael to apologize for the way I had treated him, to try to begin some ritual of forgiveness that might clear the clouds.

In return Michael let me in on the secret of his anguish about leaving Nancy. She had been raped by her boss at a Christmas party while drunk and yet would not leave her job, as she didn't feel she could get any other. She guffawed at the idea of legal complaint, refused counseling, and lingered over but rejected Michael's offers to kill the guy. Instead, she ate herself sick and gained a hundred pounds in a year, withdrew from any social life, and went blank. Michael said he had been unable to reach her in two years of trying, but the guilt of departing—and of deceiving me about it—had snaked around him, all through him, with a stranglehold he had taken years to loosen. No wonder we had not survived as a couple.

Blown away by my own blindness, I bumbled my way home after this conversation, realizing once again the extent of my delusions. Here I had convinced myself that I needed to go back to the end of my relationship with Michael in order to ferret out the source of the toxins, but of course that fountain flowed much earlier—to the beginning of my relationship with Michael, even further back to Tom, to Rod, to the lonely years of high school. Maybe it went even further back than my diabetes, maybe my diabetes didn't necessarily create that fountain, but I kept finding traces of my illness in the poisonous effluents, diabetes feeding the stream of my insecurities, seeping into the pool of dark dreams I encountered in others, spewing up bubbles of rotten love.

When years later I received the news that Nancy, at the age of forty, had died of a massive cerebral hemorrhage, the guilty shock entered my bone marrow more quickly than when Michael had told me of her rape; the surprise filtered out in a matter of minutes to leave only sorrow and a renewed sense of the unintelligibility of the universe. It should have been *me* dying early of a stroke, I thought. That happens to *diabetics*, not to normal, healthy people. In a way, she and I seemed to have changed places, traded fates, or at least merged and confused them. Yet I had never known her, had only seen photos of her, taken during the early years of her marriage to Michael—she slender and tanned, one limber leg bent and pulled up, her firm heel hooked over the edge of the chair, the warm vitality of her beautiful eyes shining toward the camera. Once optimistic and alive, now gone. I knew that in my own quest for love and affirmation, I had contributed to her death, and this has led me a little ways toward forgiveness of Bill. And my diabetes—it is the same—I must love the disease for what it has taught me, without thinking that it is what I deserve. I cannot wish my disease away, as it permeates my self completely now. Instead, I try to learn its preferences like those of any spouse, to coddle and indulge it like any favorite, to understand the secrets it shares with me, to value its constant, deepening companionship all the way to the grave: my diabetes, the lover that will never leave me, the one I think of all the time, the only one that penetrates me to my soul.

part three

A Knot of
Chocolate-Covered
Pretzels

In a long northwestern veer they burst out into
Pennsylvania, wondering if it would be cooler as the
sun sank. . . . Not too fast, Clegg told Booth. "In
Pennsylvania they fine you a dollar for every mile per
hour over the limit."

—Paul West, *Terrestrials*

I n these long days of summer, I sit here at my computer, up high
on the second floor of my townhouse perched on the apex of a
hill that slopes away covered all around with trees and homes. Of
a Saturday, dusk may fall as I write and keep on writing into the
evening. I have no plans: no date, no party to go to, no movie to
see, no dinner invitation. I will continue to plunk the keys until
darkness blankets thickly around me and I am tired enough to
sleep.

Mostly I am content, but tonight, as on many nights during
the summer, I can hear a gathering of people at one of the houses
below me on the hillside. Voices burble and rise, then subside
into a murmur of private story-sharing between bouts of laughter, remonstrances to the children, and the occasional whoop
or booming objection. As the young splash in the kiddie pool
and thunder across the yard and deck, I become attuned to my

separation. Though I can see the screen in front of me, I cannot see or touch or participate in that peaceful weekend. Only in memory and imagination do I feel the pool's now-tepid water, see the sparkle of wetness flung through the air and caught in the spokes of moon or citronella candle, smell the way the dampness of the whirling children's hair invokes the trace of baby shampoo from their warm scalps. Only memory and imagination still bind me to all that I am missing right now: close family, easy companionship, constant connection.

Yet I love this room where I am sitting. Beyond my computer screen the window fills with the murky blue of twilight, its square occupied half by the silhouettes of three massive evergreens and one ancient apple tree, half by the fading clouds and reviving silver moon. To my left, a bulletin board crammed with photos of friends and family scattered across New York, Illinois, Tennessee, California, Minnesota, New Mexico, Massachusetts, Virginia; a tall bookcase, also crowded to its edges; and my great-grandmother's Sheffield bureau, its rat-holed drawers now filled with manila folders and check registers, office supplies and teaching files. On the right, before another window, two huge plants soak up the day's sun, and a long table (actually a door atop two file cabinets) stretches the length of the wall under a large poster of South America, where I hope someday to travel. Behind that, another bookshelf and a poster of Laurel Falls in the Great Smokies, where I have often been and hope to return. Usually, my old cat sleeps in the extra chair, every now and then lifting her head, blinking her green eyes at me, and purring for a few moments before her pink nose nods back down to her paws. Sometimes, however, she likes to secrete herself behind a file box or a stack of books in the maze of papers and tomes that lines the room all around. In addition to the door–file cabinet table and the Sheffield chest, the room contains three bookcases, a wooden card table, a computer table, a drafting table, two office chairs, two lamps, a printer, and two computers, and yet it functions without seeming cramped. For such a tiny room, this one holds an amazing assortment of flora and fauna, places far and near, faces, air, and ideas.

Often financially strapped, I think about getting a housemate, but I cannot face giving up this room. I am greedy for space, for the quiet that allows my thoughts to grow unchecked, not interrupted by others' expectations and needs. The last housemate I had here, who occupied this room, blew his nose like a freight-train whistle, listened in on my phone conversations, and spattered the kitchen with grease and beef blood that he never seemed to notice. Here, in this dear room, the smell of his long-unwashed gym clothes hung in the air of every warm day until I plastered the inside of the closet with stick-up deodorant disks. Eradicating all traces of him brought me great pleasure, a sense of self-possession, and a stunning peace.

Still, I thought living by myself would be a fairly brief phase. I told my departing housemate and my friends that I had just reached an age where it seemed impossible to share such small spaces with someone I didn't really know and love. I assumed that someone, whether friend or paramour, would meet my criteria soon enough. Now nearly eight years have passed, as though magical invisible bricks have flown in from nowhere to fill up the doorways and windows, more and more solidly closing me in here. Like a nun in black, like a cloistered sister, her stiff skirts impeding her stride, the rosary in her waist swaying in reminder, head sometimes swimming with possibility but calmed by the prospect of work, the balm of never-ending labor, and the firm walls closing her in with her own mind, to her own god, I pace the limits of my apartment.

When I leave the study, I have three choices. I can go straight, then left down the stairs, or I can turn right into the bathroom, with its cerulean and pink tiles and the window in the shower that allows me to bathe in the sunlight and the breezes of summer (ah, the illusions thus created—that I wash under a waterfall, that I live in the fresh air, that the rain is always warm, that the world is not ruined . . .). Or I can bear far left into the bedroom, where I love the way the light flickers through the birch tree outside and plays across the bed, turning the blocks of the quilt into a perfect smooth-and-jagged, yin-yang, both beauteously terrifying and meltingly peaceful complement of measured square and fluttery irregular leaf tangling like so many emotions and bodies in my private space. For someone so immured, I certainly am fond of what creeps and leaps through the glass from outside. It forms a large portion of all the dialogue that is available here in this silent, spoken-wordless place, though of course I talk out loud with the cat and the telephone, and speechlessly through my typing.

Upstairs and downstairs, however, one might say that I also converse these days with the history of the objects, my past, dead and gone people who have helped constitute myself. Almost every item here embodies a story, and I can tell you the source and cause of virtually every one of them; if they suddenly arrayed themselves in chronological order, I suppose there would be no need to write a life story—it would be laid out for all to see, for me to understand. As it is, they are all jumbled up, the polyester blocks of the quilt pieced by my Grandmother Roney covering the late-model floral sheets picked out by my father's second wife, and both adorning the cherry bed my mother's parents had made in Gatlinburg. This, even though my father horrified his own mother by divorcing mine much as my Grandfather Roney had divorced her forty years earlier, even though my mother's parents most certainly would never have forgiven him—here they all meet again, all around my bed, where I myself have merged and wrestled with men and books and hypoglycemic monsters that none of them would approve.

Downstairs, my great-grandmother Irene's blue pottery biscuit bowl nests more companionably inside another heavy dish given to me by a grad-school friend. The yellow chairs from a college dining hall where my grandparents ate cluster around the table I picked out myself years later, a table alternately piled high with mail and papers, burdened with pots of herbs and African violets (which I'm trying to learn to grow as my grandfather did assiduously), scattered with candlesticks I never bothered to return to a guy named Pete, the crystal vase from Panos, and my favorite childhood wooden blocks, which I use as paperweights, but which properly aligned form the loveliest mutated creatures, part frog, part bear, part chicken, part rabbit. These might have been my mother's before they were my brother's and mine, but my memory does not go back that far.

All my lovers' photos, those not in the landfill, keep each other company in a series of albums on the same shelf. No one is jealous anymore, except perhaps me.

On the walls downstairs there is a watercolor by my uncle, a tiny print by my old friend Susan, a madeleine pan from my writer friend Sally in honor of Proustian prose, a flattened trumpet that I found at a party with Michael, and the funny little cat-faced mirror I bought in Philadelphia when I visited Melanie a couple of years ago. The bathroom walls sport art postcards, collected in my college days, of people in various stages of undress, company for those getting into the shower, and the kitchen walls, a plethora of food postcards, including a pic of the side of a thirties diner advertising BRAINS, 25¢. I wish the price were still so reasonable.

Cradled in my apartment are more than a thousand books in

eight bookcases, nine hundred postcards (antique and contemporary), a mere fifty-nine CDs and forty-nine tapes, but a hundred and fifty fine pieces of vinyl, fifty-some-odd jars of spices, thirty-three potted plants (fourteen outside on the porches), about thirty T-shirts, twenty-five volumes of my journal, twenty-three pairs of shoes, twenty-two skirts and fifteen dresses (several of which I haven't worn in a few seasons), sixteen flavors of tea, eleven unmatched coffee mugs, seven or eight handmade quilts in various states of wear, seven varieties of skin lotion for my itchy legs, six (unopened) condoms, six bottles of insulin (three unopened, three in use), six bottles of pills (none unopened), five types of flour, four embroidered pillowcases, three each of English-language dictionaries, kinds of shampoo, and iron skillets, two telephones, two frozen chicken breasts, two jugs of white grape juice, two coffee grinders (one hand-cranked, one electrical), two candlesticks, two tablecloths (one a gargantua, made by my grandmother, for that unlikely seating of twelve, and one, still seldom used, that better suits my poorly furniture), two rocking chairs, two night tables, one bed, one down comforter, one whisk, vegetable steamer, omelet pan, wok, teakettle, and toaster, one tiny television, one hammer, one squash racquet and gym bag, one glucose monitor, one set of worry beads from Greece, one cat, and the ashes of one cat. I find zero tubes of lipstick, but the multitudinous sheets of paper and the words thereon escape accountability. They multiply like dust mites.

Some days as I prowl through the house, restless and uneasy, my eyes encounter an object from the past—in it I am faced with both the long gone other person who gave it to me, or held it aloft in just such a tender way, and my perfectly alone self; that is, with the change that has overtaken me since I've come to Pennsylvania. Sometimes I marvel that no one shares this complex, peaceful, enticing, pleasant life with me. I wonder what exactly has happened to my life, so full of promise, options, all manner of exciting men and boon companions, just a few years ago. What has turned me inward—and others away? The college town doesn't particularly suit me, nor the conservative, insular quality of semi-rural Pennsylvania. My work takes a great deal of energy and attention, it excludes me from a whole realm of men who need to feel wiser, more experienced, more educated than their women, and there are plenty of sweet young things in such a town. But do ten years, ten pounds, and grad school alter so much? None of these answers seems sufficient.

It's strange, however, that in this new solitude I also find an odd familiarity even beyond the objects in my apartment. This turn inward, away from sociability, I realize, happened long ago, but has just now captured my fleeing stride. I have only now, perhaps, turned and embraced a shadow running behind me for years, the aftermath of a strange adolescence, the sentence of an untimely death. How fantastical to know what will be the cause of one's death when one is twelve! Even if that death is not the one that comes, all manner of unacceptable prescience comes with the named possibility, all kinds of burdens that one's peers will understand only when they are sixty, and maybe not even then.

In the years immediately following my diagnosis, I had the melancholy habit of lying on the carpeted floor in front of the stereo speakers, facedown, listening over and over to the tunes of Simon and Garfunkel—"Kathy's Song," "The Boxer," "Sounds of Silence," "Old Friends," "Scarborough Fair." Many an afternoon after school, I would go directly there and sprawl, sometimes with the warmth of my dog curled beside me, until my mother got home and rallied me for setting the table or making the salad.

Granted, many a nondiabetic kid has done such, but now in my mind I go back there, very definitely there—it is those moments that make my current life familiar in spite of its newness. Perhaps my illness only gives me a retrospective excuse for a personality I would have had no matter what. The thing is that I will never know. I only know that I have spent years pretending not to be all alone with it, pretending that it did not set me apart. Other kids are alienated by other aspects of their painful lives, and diabetes doesn't alienate all children who get it, but that's what it did for me. My family and friends and doctors and I called it everything else: stubbornness, anti-authoritarianism, feminism, sexual freedom, love troubles, political outrage, intellectual independence, man-hating, experimentation, selfishness, workaholism, perfectionism, when, really, I was just trying to find a socially acceptable way not to fit in, perhaps some marginal niche where I would belong.

But chronic illness is too individual for that, too particular and varied. The separateness is carried by the absolute individuality of the body, its capacities and limits. Both curse and the necessary condition of survival, both self and not-self, the arcane requirements of illness cannot be shared, often even among those with the same illness. In this way, there are differences from other kinds of marginal communities—gay and lesbian, feminist, Rainbow people, and so on. We, the ill, are dictated to by our bodies, not our minds, and each of us handles it differently, finds different boundaries and balances, with nuances making incredible differences in our lives.

In other words, even if illness were generally socially acceptable, or if I filled my life with diabetics, I would still need to retreat every now and then, to sleep my extra fill, to regulate my diet and exercise, and to perform the private rituals of my disease.

Being a writer—of memoir, of dissertation—is in many ways ideal, and lately has given me a great degree of control over my own schedule. I can adjust my exercise to my blood sugar levels without any problem, can sleep extra if I've had a bad low, can for the most part maintain a time-consuming and amazingly regular routine. Sometimes I vary this routine according to another person's schedule—a late lunch with a friend, a party that goes on through the night—but few people realize the toll this can take on me if I try to get by with too much of it, and this goes even for people with whom I have lived. I have never lived so peacefully and regularly with someone else in the house. In this regard the solitude is not my enemy.

However, it unnerves me to border on the phenomenon I refer to as "diabetic Puritanism," a kind of conservatism for its own sake that pervades much of the medical and diabetic-community discourse about how best to live with the disease. Recently, in reading up on lotions for my typically sensitive and fragile diabetic skin, I came across a couple of articles in recent for-diabetics publications suggesting particular products and qualities; one of the latter was that a lotion be unscented. Suspicious, I asked my doctor, "Short of unrelated allergies, is there any reason why diabetics shouldn't use sweet-smelling lotion?"

"Nope," he said.

"More of that diabetic Puritanism?" I guessed.

"I suppose so," he nodded.

Why, I fumed, with all the other (real and necessary) restrictions on our physical pleasures, should these publications be denying us this one? It gives me a simple, little trivial joy to be complimented on my habitual vanilla scent, to put my nose against my arm and breathe in something nonmedicinal, to participate in the universe of the body beautiful—so often so far from me. And yet there is a whole raft of these disgusting special products advertised—hideous orthotically correct shoes, ugly white seamless socks to prevent blisters, bizarre tools for examining the feet, odious vinyl pouches for carrying supplies, foul food products that may not contain sugar but will make you gassy. Not that some or all of these items aren't useful and don't answer real needs. Sigh. But they are also constant reminders of one's medicalized state, and they and the advice that comes with them often go too far in separating us from the run of life.

In last December's issue of the American Diabetes Association magazine, an article on coping with the overabundance of holiday goodies at social events recommended that you sit down with a list of all your party invitations and decide which ones you could just avoid. Great, huh? To prevent overeating, just stay home. Do we really have to isolate ourselves this way in order to live at all? Unfortunately, to a certain extent the answer is yes—and this is the hardest thing to face—but the exact location of that boundary line is uncertain, variable, a constant locus of negotiation. It is incredibly hard to balance enjoying life by indulgence and enjoying it by a rigorously maintained health regimen.

One thing that contributes to the difficulty of this is the general direction of society these days—toward "tolerance," which means, among other, often positive things, a lack of common standards for behavior and levels of self-indulgence. There exists no longer a common dinner hour, or a dinner hour at all, or even an expectation that someone will eat dinner. That fact in itself presents incredible difficulties for diabetics, but multiply it by all the other aspects of daily life to which the variations now apply, and it becomes a morass. Combine it with a general attitude of instant gratification as the norm, and social interaction looms a downright demon on the horizon of every day.

When I was child, I adored chocolate-covered pretzels. All year long I anticipated the single box we would buy at Christmastime, two dozen medium-sized pretzels sitting prettily in the individual slots of the plastic packaging nestled in the long, pale blue rectangular container, as festive to me as any red-and-green decorations. One department store, Miller's, carried these special confections only during the holiday season, and it was a ritual stop on my family's earliest shopping trips. We meted them out, one by one, over the month of December, their smooth, rich cocoa like the warm mud of spring over the salty crustiness of pretzels and the crisp, ice-coated ground of winter. They perfected the time of year, kept it in perspective, represented the hope of the rotating seasons and the balance of opposites. As such a rarity, they produced no conflicts.

Now, in my local grocery store, on any given day of any given week, I can find at least three varieties of chocolate-covered pretzel: the huge, dollar-apiece ones sold individually at the gourmet coffee counter; the cheap, waxy variety sold in plastic bags in the nut aisle; and the new, expensive Nestlé brand in bright, gaudy foil bags in the candy racks. I still like them, and it is now completely up to me to regulate my consumption, to say "not now," to pass them by as they reach out with a hundred other available fabulous treats telling me that I deserve to have whatever I want at every possible moment of each day. Now each pretzel queries me, "Is it worth it to eat me? Will the melting sweetness on your tongue, the satisfying crunch between your teeth, make up for the potential damage to your eyes, the frustrating leap in your glucose readings, in the sluggish way you may feel tomorrow?" Perhaps, in addition to staying home from holiday parties, I should avoid the grocery store, but instead I spend gadzooks of dollars on fresh strawberries, which I love as much, but which don't do the same number on my blood sugar.

Still, these chocolate-covered pretzels tie knots in my stomach as a symbol of how I've tried to lead a "normal" life, over and over desiring to be and acting like "everybody else" (as though it would be okay for anyone to eat a steady diet of candy). Gradually, over the years after I left home for college, I behaved less and less like a sick person, and what great relief there was in that, at least for a time. Still, I had been speeding, squandering my energy in flurries of misdirected activity. Sooner or later, one pays a heavy fine for this kind of life—later for the generally healthy, sooner for me. Here in Pennsylvania, it caught up to me, and I've had to refigure the balance by myself.

Alone, our minds (and souls, if you will) may still go anywhere in any company—converse, argue, shout, make love, and cross oceans—but we can be truly alone with our bodies, those things we can't see without a mirror, without the approval or approbation of someone else. So, now, more than anything else, I am trying to learn how to understand my body on its own terms, including the coming end, the temporary nature of this physical existence patched together by doctors, researchers, sacrificial dogs and cows and pigs, by my own continual effort. This body's beauties and horrors are largely invisible to anyone else, and perhaps they even fall outside our usual descriptive categories. There is no beauty, there is no ugliness, there is no strength or weakness, superiority or inferiority. Comparisons are moot; there is just this body full of blood and bones, covered by a canvas of skin, walking toward a certain future at an uncertain time.

For now, provisionally, I labor my way away from being a victim in that inevitable, comparative world, trying not to be psychically twisted by an illness that renders me competitively inferior in a society obsessed by success, by the need to hide my own vulnerability and need, to overcompensate for the burden that I am. Does the distance between me and those relaxed families at the house down the hill indicate that I am failing? Or that I am succeeding on my own terms, based upon the limitations I am trying to face, to really face?

Raised to value at least the appearance of lack of need, if the real unilateral self-sufficiency is impossible, I am good at living alone, at forging ahead, at focusing on my work, at taking joy where I may find it. Typical of my friends, my old high school comrade Susan, who struggles to balance her practice as an artist with her close family life—nearby parents, siblings, in-laws, nieces and nephews, as well as her own husband and son—tells me she admires and envies how "fiercely independent" I am.

Independent, yes, but the only thing that is fierce is the loneliness.

8

Mild, Little Nightmares

Kay and I sat on opposite sides of her desk, face to face, both staring, though she could probably not see that I did and she probably did not know that she did. She smiled and talked, but her pale eyes did not move across my burning face. I felt as though I were looking into some kind of strange mirror of my future, or a picture like Dorian Gray's, or an abyss. Yet I kept telling myself to get a grip, asking myself what was wrong with me, hoping that my intestines would quit writhing in my gut, cursing my lack of sympathy, the pure horror and fear which I'd thought I was above. But there was something about Kay that frightened me: about my age and a diabetic for about the same duration, she was almost stone blind from diabetic retinopathy.

At thirty-one, with much trepidation and uncertainty about whether or not I could manage it, I had gone back to school full-time to pursue an M.F.A. in fiction writing. If few people with handicaps and chronic illnesses finish bachelor's degrees, our numbers in graduate school are miniscule. The first semester, between taking demanding courses and teaching my own class of freshman composition, racing between home and campus on foot, climbing the stacks in the library, staying up late to finish writing or grading papers, reading hundreds of pages a week, and attending evening lectures and readings, I thought I would simply die. My body ached continuously as though it had been pounded with an oversized meat mallet. My brain rattled against my skull with insecurity and eyestrain, and my dinners went from home-cooked and healthy to bags of microwave popcorn tossed with Parmesan cheese scarfed down while I crouched over a book or stack of papers. My savings account dwindled rapidly, as it had to pay for emergency car repairs and doctor appointments as well as the expensive books my courses required, and at the end of that first semester I had to ask my nosy, noisy, and bad-smelling housemate to move out. Broke, and ashamed to be back on the parental dole, I sought extra funding wherever I could. Someone had told me that there were several scholarships for medical expenses available through the university's Office of Disability Services, and so I had gone by one day to pick up an application. An advisor there, Kay was helping me apply for medical-expense scholarship money.

I found myself completely unprepared for my reaction to Kay, and I sorrowed over it. After all, I had worked for almost a year as a study assistant to a young woman who was going blind from a hereditary condition, and this had never bothered me in the least. I was frightened in Kay by the proximity of the blindness, a kind of blindness that I had dreaded since my diagnosis, but which I had shoved to the far corners of my mind. I had rendered it a non-issue, an unreal possibility, as remote as Afghanistan.

Now, sitting across from Kay, it came back with all the force of a missile aimed directly at me, even though I should have known better. Did I want to classify myself as disabled in order to get a few hundred dollars? I had never done so before, and the label, frankly, scared me.

For once, too, the question arose as to "Why not me? How have I escaped the worst so far?" Certainly over the years I had contemplated its inverse—Why me? Why did I get diabetes? What did I do to deserve this?—and in fact I simply don't believe people who claim they don't feel that way about their life-threatening diseases. It seems to me to be the most natural question in the world to ask when something dreadful has befallen you, and asking it does not necessarily render you an unrelenting whiner. Some time later, when I was reintroduced to Kay at a meeting of diabetic college students, she commented herself, upon comparing our similar ages and dissimilar conditions, that I must have been "awfully good," that she-hadn't-been-and-see-where-it-had-gotten-her. This struck me as tragic—self-blame for the ravages of a terrible condition—whether she had actually behaved less "properly" than I or not, and I squirmed in her presence once again. One of the reasons was that, upon my first meeting with her, I had wondered, Why not me? I knew that the main answer was "Luck," but luck is such a thin ice upon which to glide, on which to know that your sight, your kidney function, your life depend, suspended over that deep, frigid water below.

We all want to have gotten the rewards of our lives because we deserve them somehow, because we have earned them, and yet the flip side is that we must deserve as well the ills that befall us. We live in a society founded upon the idea that everyone should get what he or she deserves, and it really is a nation where there is more flexibility than usual in terms of class and accomplishment, but not even the most egalitarian government can render life fair. We are so in the habit of believing that the rich have merited their money, that movie stars and athletes were born superior, and that a fancy car equates significantly with manhood that we forget how this punishes us—for our close-to-the-margin bank accounts, our own extra ten pounds, and the fact that our perfume does not cost $300 an ounce. With stronger and stronger realizations of this dark side of merit, I tend to believe less and less in causation. If I go blind, I will refuse the added burden of blaming myself for that.

My doctor says that no one who attends as closely as I do to my diabetes goes blind, but every time I eat a cookie I wonder if this is the one that will push me over the edge to culpability. Am I doing as well as Dr. Ulbrecht thinks I am, as I appear to be? Or is this just another way that I have people fooled? Haven't I partaken of plenty of coconut chip ice cream, Godiva chocolate, buttered bread, and sticky buns? The line between good enough and not good enough is pretty blurry. It is not that I want to deny the critical difference good control can make to long-term diabetic health, but I remain stubborn on this point. Kay, I insist, is not blind because of some flaw in her eating habits; she is blind because diabetes is a cruel and devastating illness that wreaks havoc on the entire body and breaks it down bit by bit, part by part, organ by organ, affecting not only eyes but ears, brain, gums, mucous membranes, heart, kidneys, intestines, and all the minute nerves and blood vessels that reach to the genitals, the fingertips, the toes. Sometimes it does this quickly, sometimes slowly, and statistically it is true that the closer to normal you keep your blood sugar, the better your chances are of slowing it; but the fact is that there are no guarantees and some lives and some bodies are easier to keep in line than others. The effects are there in all of us, just as death waits in every living body every-where.

The latter, of course, is what people want to deny when they blame the ill for their conditions. If your own bad behavior is to blame, then it will never happen to them. Countless times during my childhood and adolescence, when told of my diabetes, people would snidely state, "You get that from eating too much sugar, don't you." No question mark, no room for a rebuttal, for if you rebut that just means you are making excuses.

Over the years, I've tried various strategies in answer to this statement, most often merely saying, "No, you don't," and speaking in a tone of voice that indicates my authority. I've also tried acknowledging what small truth there might be in this belief by explaining that there are two kinds of diabetes and that it's only Type 2 that correlates at all with overeating. Just a few days ago, buying new running shoes, when I explained that diabetes made me somewhat stiff in the ankles, the salesclerk proceeded to tell me all about his diabetic father, who had lost a hundred pounds after being diagnosed and taking up a rigorous exercise program. "How fat were you to begin with?" he seemed to be asking, but he said, "He's even got off insulin. Maybe you can, too." When I told him I had the other kind of diabetes, he had no idea what I meant. So, even when I revert to my own version of the idea that some people may deserve it, but that I don't, it does me little good, seldom getting through to my audience. Their faces usually glaze over thick as that milky sugar on a donut, and sometimes I fantasize about leaning over and biting the dumpling-smooth cheeks of those who ignore my explanations. I've tried to place myself with the blameless and only end up face-to-face with a human dessert shut off from me. So there, I say in my fantasy, is it your fault that I've bitten your willfully naïve face off?

Nowadays I usually tell people that it is an autoimmune disease, but this doesn't work very well either, as people have grown to believe that if they take the right vitamins their own immune systems will be strong and pure. My reply becomes to them just a fancy way of saying that I ate too much sugar, that I somehow destroyed my own immune system. When I tell people that my mother had kept me on an incredibly healthy diet—that my first refined sugar was my first birthday cake, that we only had candy at holidays, that we never drank soda—the response changes, and the medieval paradigm of homeopathy prevails. I must've got diabetes because my body never learned to handle sugar. Me or my mother, either of us will do for the blame. Few really take an interest in the biochemical and causal complexities—they want a simple reason that leaves them out of it.

Yet I can no longer condemn this evasive fear—or even that of the most obtuse and unkind—for when I first encountered Kay's blindness, so close to my own eyes and yet a world of experience away, I felt the same longing for a reason, for assurance that it would not, could not, be me.

Recently I thought of Kay again, when my ophthalmologist gently announced to me that he could see the beginnings of cataracts growing in the depths of my eyes. Retinopathy still minimal, but cataracts already showing. "It will be some years yet before they affect your sight," he said, "and, of course, when they do, they are eminently treatable. They just tend to become a problem for diabetics at age fifty instead of the normal seventy."

At home later, lying on the couch, staring at the blank, blank ceiling, I recalled Kay with her dog and cane, her talking computer and watch, and I wondered about the progressive falling of her dominoes—first the diabetes, then the proliferative retinopathy, the kidney trouble she had more recently mentioned.

Diabetes is like this: one loss after another, year after year, with constant anticipation of more, a narrowing path of health and activity. We are sitting ducks waiting for the complications to arrive, one by one. You can never quite adjust to the disease because it is always changing, always staking out another province in some new part of the body, stealthily, with all the silence of the worms waiting underground. In such a circumstance, of course, one fears most of all oneself.

In the year after my diagnosis, lying down to go to sleep, night after night, I would grow afraid. I suffered from recurring nightmares, all centering on death and savagery. These dreams were graphic in a way that still shocks me when I recall my innocence at the time. I had seen only Uncle Russell's dead body, though I would see several more at open-casket funerals in the next couple of years. I had never watched a movie rated R for its violence (or anything else). I had grown up in quiet suburbs where kids still played outside without their parents' direct supervision. My nightmares reflected a reality that I couldn't have known about, except in some Jungian collective or mythic sense. Or perhaps in the sense that my body already knew what my mind was in the process of discovering.

In one of these dreams, the one that recurred most frequently and that still recurs from time to time in variation, I am at home with my family—both my parents, brother, grandparents, sometimes aunts, uncles, and cousins. Usually we are sitting at the dinner table—ours was a big round of oak that sat in front of a picture window—when the shooting begins. Of course, it takes us by surprise, and a couple of us are always killed right away, window glass shattering and blood flying into the air, spattering the paint and wood, limp bodies suddenly in the way of escape.

Over the course of the dream, everyone is picked off, one by one, until I am left alone in the house, crawling along the floor hugging the walls underneath the windows, through the broken debris that was my life. When I glimpse the sniper, he is always in the same position, dressed in hunting garb and aiming a rifle my way. But he never moves when I see him, as though a still photograph, a frozen image of evil and threat. In the world of dream interpretation, a home represents the self. Mine certainly came under attack in my sleeping life, and, while I never die in this dream—and there have been hundreds of variations over the years—I creep in circles of terror, knowing there is no way to escape alive.

The other nightmare occurred only a few times shortly after my diagnosis. But I remember it vividly, literally as though I dreamed it last night. In it, I am with my two dear friends, sisters nicknamed Mouse and Barndoor, and we are already afraid, have been captured, and are together in some dark, endless space without walls—the way a dark scene on a stage appears. We cannot see our captors, as they are dressed in black, wear masks, and blind us with spotlights, but they have heavy, cruel voices like the sound of trucks grinding their gears. They give Mouse a rifle and tell her that if she doesn't shoot us, then in front of her they will torture us until we die. Together we agonize over this, and finally decide that she should do it—what other choice do we have? We are more worried about leaving Mouse there than about dying. What will they do to her once we are gone? Why have they chosen her for the difficult job? Who is doing this to us anyway, and why? What have we done? We don't really want to die without some explanation.

Finally, though, the pressure is on, the men are shouting and gesticulating, and Mouse shoots, first me—and I have the classic sensation of rising like a ghost from my body and floating above the scene looking down. I see Mouse shoot Barndoor, and I see Barndoor's self also rising. She and I find that we can talk without talking, and we float there, worried about Mouse, who is moaning and crying in disbelief at what she's done. She makes a wailing inhuman noise, part animal but mostly industrial—like a foghorn, a steam turbine whine, finally the squeal before a car accident. The scene below is one of horror, and Barndoor and I look on, the worst thing being that there's nothing we can do. Death isn't physically painful to us, but it is frustratingly incapacitating.

Always there, looking down, I would awaken, shaking, unsure in my dark bedroom which side of the reality-dream line I was on. Usually I had already called out, and my mother would soon come and smooth my forehead until I calmed down and went back to sleep. We never considered these nightmares a symptom of a desperate sense of living under siege, of losing everything. We never talked about them in the daylight.

A few pages into my first journal, begun the summer after I graduated from high school, I write, "I am feeling better, at least I am able to stay relatively cheerful. It's such a bother to act depressed around this household because everyone makes such a big thing out of it." I complained in the same way of my new friends at college. Clearly, it was I who was out of step, and clearly it was an effort for me to maintain a socially acceptable level of sanguinity. By college, this had been going on for years. "What do you have to be depressed about?" one of my friends wrote to me the fall I was twelve. I wonder how I answered her. In those early letters, I wonder, where is diabetes, where is muscle wastage, where urinating every fifteen minutes, where the forbidden nature of ice cream, where the warnings to boys I might date, where the muddled thought process, where the sentence including blindness and children with birth defects and daily needles in my flesh and early death?

Depression affects nearly a quarter of all people with diabetes, and it is twice as common among diabetics as among the general population, but health care professionals seldom raise the topic, at least in my experience. You have to bring it up yourself somehow, something that is virtually impossible for a child—with little perspective and no worldly experience—to do. For me, instead, the depression went underground, and pooled there like a great, growing aquifer, soaking up the rainwater without ever a release. I am convinced that the depths of my depression could have been prevented had I only understood what it was.

As it happened, I developed a strong resonance, not so much with the insane or otherwise "disturbed" themselves, but with social commentary that viewed the psychic responses of those labeled mentally ill as often appropriate in the face of a warped world and that even sometimes expressed a cartload of rage against the idea that we should all remain "normal," no matter the circumstances. Somewhere in the middle range in terms of my ability and willingness to normalize my difficulties, I nonetheless sympathize with those who do not. The extremely well-adjusted do not even need my respect—they get enough from those who use them to prove that "we are all alike," that handicaps are something to be overcome. I spent years silently angry, and then read a book called *The Survivor: An Anatomy of Life in the Death Camps*, about Holocaust-survivor psychology. I wept with recognition. Even though the pains of my own experience do not compare to the horror of a death camp, never in any cheerful, helpful book on chronic illness or diabetes had I read anything that made so much sense to me about myself. The book's exploration of the survivor's need and driving will to tell the story, the confrontation with disgusting aspects of physical existence, a capacity for realism, the strange renewal of life in the continual face of possible death—I found myself in these patterns. It was the first moment that I allowed myself to form the conscious thought that I might have something to be *legitimately* less than happy about. I was more than thirty years old.

Already, I had been in therapy off and on for several years, beginning when I was twenty-three and sleeping with a married man and my father announced that he was leaving my mother for another woman. My diabetes had seldom been the topic of that therapy or even acknowledged as the permanent subtext of my daily life. Instead, my first, very ineffective shrink listened to me complain—about my boyfriend, about my father, about my colleagues and the demeaning stupidity of my job, about my own lack of direction and my uncertainty about what I wanted to do with my life. The only feedback she gave was to restate what I'd just said in classic reflective language, and she yawned a lot during our sessions, hiding this by not allowing her mouth to open fully, but with her nostrils flaring in telltale symptom. I might as well have been talking to the wind, and the process did very little for me, though there was no doubt that I needed help.

I had acquired my shrink not by recommendations from friends but by bursting into tears "for no reason" in my physician's office after he told me how well I was doing with my diabetes after all those years. No one, I realized, had ever told me that, and virtually no one had ever praised me for anything except not letting it "get in the way." At my tears, the doctor hastily shipped me around the corner to the therapist who practiced in the cut-rate clinic associated with the hospital where he practiced. He told her that my love life was troubled, but my diabetes remained buried.

Admittedly, it was a phase when I cried at almost anything. Watching the movie *Sybil*—about a girl who suffers from multiple personality disorder after having been abused by her mother— I sobbed uncontrollably, a reaction so strong and bizarre that I wondered incredulously if it were possible I had been abused myself. A few weeks later, however, I performed the same trick while sitting in front of a Benji-the-dog movie wherein a nice family is injured in a car crash and the pup is lost in the desert in all the hubbub of getting the people to the hospital. I even cried at *Gremlins*, a comedy in which one little monster gets scrambled in a food processor. I could hardly listen to any kind of music without trembling, my heart bruising on every melancholy note.

The moment in the doctor's office, however, probably was the first time I had cried only for myself, in pure indulgent self-pity and longing. I had no idea what I was doing, but I would begin to find out.

Throughout the years I have also cycled through two other regularly recurring types of dreams—these vary in terms of situation and fellow passengers, but they can be grouped into "fighting" and "paralysis" dreams. In the latter, I am attacked, usually physically, and freeze, unable to make a sound. Many people dream of falling—in front of rushing trains or cars—and being unable to stand or move, but I have never had that type of dream; rather, what races toward me is always another person, a violent and enormous man, and the horror is that I cannot speak or scream. Instead, my voice itself chokes me, transmuting in my own throat into a material clog, the water backing up behind it as though to drown me. My chest expands as though filling with filthy fluid and feels as though it will explode, but time stops. The attacker never hurts me, and my hammering heart does not achieve a crack in my torso through which blood and water might flood out. It is only that I am afraid and silent and can find no words or sounds with which to tell.

The fighting dreams embarrass me, I suppose because I worry that they are too true, or that they represent some reality about me that is unpleasant. Most of them are trivial, daily life–based situations in which I am yelling at my co-workers, or my family, or my current or ex-boyfriend, or some such hapless person, always someone that I'm in waking life angry with but to whom my explanations seem ignored or misunderstood. In the dream, every witness's face expresses that I am overreacting to something and they think I'm crazy. Still, they are ashamed, and I find this effect beautifully rewarding, as though they have finally gotten the point. These are dreams of guilty pleasure, though when I awaken I languish, saddened at the fact that my honest expression is so damaging, that this streak of violent anger runs alongside my terrified silence.

It is difficult to speak the truth of illness. Half the time, those of us who are ill don't even have a sense of what is real and what is illusion created by hope or by the intervention of the healthy protecting themselves. In a recent diabetic newsletter there ran an emotional debate about the implications of using "diabetic" versus "a person with diabetes." The argument goes that the latter is better because it doesn't imply that the diabetes defines you, but is merely one aspect of your life. Now, I'm an English teacher, a writer, and a hair-splitter in terms of vocabulary and syntax, but I believe this debate was created by diabetes educators—and that those who consider "diabetic" an evil label feel demeaned by it only because some nurse practitioner told them they should. Do you feel put down by being called a baker or a lawyer, rather than a person who bakes or a person who practices law? Of course not, because everyone understands that those labels are context specific and partial, just as is "diabetic." On the other hand, do you feel any better about "a person who molests children" than you do about a "child molester"? Of course not. But many diabetics have taken this added burden on themselves, thinking of a word that is inevitably applied to them as a negative label, and all because someone tried to think of a kinder, sweeter way of speaking of us.

I have no patience with this euphemistic sense of the world. In that same newsletter, a story ran about a diabetic man who had been confused with a drunk and had been beaten up by the police. A woman, mother of a diabetic child, wrote that she didn't want to hear such negative things. What she wants is a publication that stays optimistic, that will cheer her up. My reaction to her is one of anger and of identification with her child, who will grow up disallowed from his fear and anguish. I needn't worry: it will emerge somehow someday. But I hate for him to have to wait twenty years, as I did, to begin to come to grips with the depth of the pain of not being normal. It takes a lot of courage to face it, but sooner or later one must. One's dreams—of choking, of shouting—will only do for so long. Inevitably, we have to speak, even if no one really wants to listen, even if what we say makes no conventional sense.

For some years I transferred onto psychotherapy my desire to be cured. My diabetes might never go away, but surely my emotional turmoil and my problematic love life could be solved and tucked away as things of the past. Since I began therapy some fifteen years ago, I have quit at least five—probably ten—times, only to be driven back again by debilitating depression—brought on by living in insane twisted caves with some boyfriend or gazing out over long, empty plains of loneliness—landscapes where I feel I do not belong, places to which I cannot trace my path once I find myself there. I have tried antidepressants now four times, and I count my numerous forays into yoga, meditation, and church as searches for this same elusive healing.

In the form of a more satisfying career, in the sense that I have a shorter tolerance for abusive friends and lovers, in a greater acceptance of my own limits and my own inability to recreate the world as I'd like it, these searches have provided enough progress through my pain that I have been at times encouraged. However, they have not granted me a cure. What I have gained instead is an understanding that nothing is really curable, which is not an understanding that any of us like particularly to have. Even many people with diabetes continue to believe the hype that has for five decades been promising a cure within five years. I never, not from the first week, subscribed to that notion, but had continued to hope in other regards—sexism, racism, poverty, alcoholism, greed, consumerism, and my own depression—that all could be reversed, ended. All of these I attacked in my therapy before ever talking of my diabetes, which emerged only gradually after years of other issues, a panoply of guises, a cornucopia of substitutes, a rainbow of distractions.

I remember when it began to dawn on me that my depression is a chronic side effect of my diabetes and unlikely ever to go away, though it has altered and will continue to alter, to shape-shift like my own spirit that underlies it all. It began in a session with my second therapist—the first worthwhile one—when I was about twenty-eight or so and mooning a bit over how none of my friends could understand what it was like to have a serious and chronic disease. My current boyfriend had told me that I used my diabetes as an excuse for being uptight when he was late for an appointment or date, and, worse, a friend had seconded him. If they thought that it was oppressive trying only occasionally to fit into the parameters of my illness, what could they possibly think about how it was for me all the time? It frustrated me that they could not even see that their freedom was a privilege—of health, of youth, of money, often of whiteness or maleness—and that I didn't have such choices to quite the same degree as they. When I complained that they didn't understand, Judy, my therapist, sagely said, "They will." I was shocked to find that what I really would have preferred was that they didn't need to understand— not that the world would eventually say no to them, but that it would quit saying no to me, that I myself could regain that delicious lack of self-consciousness and effort that comes from the juicy, flowing meld of mind and body we are born into but gradually lose to adulthood. My childhood had been so brief. I envied those attenuated ones going on around me in this adolescent-worshiping era.

But Judy was right. I now have one friend who has been on dialysis for three years, another recently diagnosed with breast cancer, several whose ideal marriages are rocking like rowboats in a gale, some who have lost or are in the process of losing parents or siblings, and too many to count who face their workdays with all the anticipation of a dog on its way to the veterinarian. I continue to find boyfriends who have never encountered a problem not of their own creation and who live with the constant illusion that they will always come out on top, but most of my friends now understand.

Yet the sensation that diabetes has been a big no, a huge rejection and punishment, has only more recently begun to fade. In my earlier therapy, I focused on self-improvement; recently I have tried for more self-acceptance. Acceptance seems such an inadequate, even flaccid word for what I mean. What I mean is so profound as to be almost indescribable, and it has to do with experiences of reality. All these years, my diabetes has presented to me, in moments, in glimpses, a reality that is seldom acknowledged by the normal world. It's not that I want to give up being a part of the regular world, but I do want to be happy with what in me is beyond that. I want to have faith in my own experience of reality, which often finds huge lacks in ordinary attitudes and beliefs.

Recently my friend Mark adopted a new dog, which had been called Cocoa at the animal shelter. He wanted to name it something that retained the *k* sound, but that would be more original. I began tossing out suggestions, as people often do in such cases, trilling off the likes of Kevin and Caleb, when Mark remarked that he had an additional challenge—his girlfriend Jennifer doesn't like to use "regular human names" for animals. Cocoa in short order became Castor, but I continued to contemplate the general acceptance of Jennifer's arbitrary preference. It was *okay* for her to insist on such a thing because she wasn't worried about fitting in, as I've always been. I have taken Jennifer as inspiration for insisting on my own perspective, of voicing my own perceptions of reality no matter how unpopular and strange they are.

One of my recent boyfriends, a sweet, smart but hapless former Deadhead, who himself was locked in a battle with the upper-class values of his lawyer father and banker mother, marveled one day that I didn't display my oddity more. "When I only knew you casually," he noted, "you seemed much less renegade. Your radicalism is so understated—I wonder why you don't play on it more, enjoy it, revel in it, show it off." Tad is right in that I probably should do so, but what he could never understand was the vast abyss between his kind of rebellion-by-choice, with a safety net, so to speak, and mine, which descended on me with all the thoroughness of a lion ripping out my guts. For me there is no going back. I cannot put on this difference and then take it off and discard it for another that feels better when the time comes. I don't really even have much choice about many of the aspects of traditional society that I accept and the ones I reject. Tad may decide he doesn't want to marry, he may choose not to wash his hair, he might opt to keep driving his father's old Volvo until he dies, he may glide from being a Deadhead through-and-through to being a graduate student to being a corporate computer engineer. Some thread of identity may even string all of these selves of his together, but they are all choices, and they can all be changed at any moment. Illness, like blackness, like femaleness, cannot. This leaves us sometimes feeling stuck, and resenting it, even if we like who we are.

Oddly, as much as I experience myself as often holding back, as trying to fit in, I have a reputation for outspokenness, which, I believe now, simply reflects how far from the usual my own perceptions of reality are. Sometimes it is hard even for me to pay attention to them, and my current therapist does not give me as much advice as my last one; rather his presence is mostly reassuring, consisting of observations without judgments, allowing me just to be the odd amalgam of aggression and timidity, independence and desperation, politeness and anger, and noncategorizable idiosyncrasy that I am. It seems a simple and perhaps silly thing to pay for, and in a moment of frustration I once said to him that it probably would have done me more good to have spent all this money on hair removal or cosmetic surgery rather than psychotherapy. No doubt had I done so, my smooth legs and my thinner face would have earned me more admiring glances—

maybe even love—than my attention to my psyche, but that, in itself, is indicative of my values. Some other people are driven to such questioning by other factors, but it is diabetes that turned me so inward and that colors my outlook now. I look out on a world that often does not welcome what or who I am, but now I am more likely to locate the poverty there than in myself.

It's not as though I have been lying on a couch for years telling Freud my dreams and having them interpreted. In fact, the content of my dreams has not been a focus of my therapy at all. I write about them here because I have noticed that my dreams follow the same kind of changing-but-staying-the-same pattern as the obsessions that have occupied my therapy. In some ways, they speak more eloquently of my struggles and transformations than any description of the banal week-to-week course of therapy ever could. During the past two years, when I've set my own schedule instead of living by a clock, in the long sleeps this has allowed—a haphazard slumber, at irregular times, interrupted by a rather calm insomnia—my dreams have become more neutral in tone, less fearful though just as odd as ever.

People move through cooked vegetables on room-sized platters, eating, talking, and tunneling through the mounds of huge slices of peppers, tomatoes, zucchini. I find it peculiar, but I shrug and begin chatting with the others there.

No longer trapped inside a house with a gunman outside, I instead climb across the terra-cotta tile roof of a long old hospital- or school-like building high atop a mountain, surrounded by mist; the roof slope is steep and the vegetation all around is dense, but I am merely concentrating on my balance without screaming or falling.

I meet a diabetic stained-glass artist named Jacob, someone I have never known in real life, and his work dazzles me with its vivid blues and yellows and its incredible precision and fragility. He says that working with glass reminds him of insulin syringes, of taking injections, which in the dream makes complete sense to me. His work, though completely nonrepresentational, is all about diabetes, and we both understand this, though it is never stated.

Most recently, I dreamed of lightning. Standing at the edge of a vast, rolling pasture surrounded by forest, I watch as a storm brews on the far, far side of the expanse. Perhaps I am one of the trees at the periphery, perhaps I am otherwise rooted to the spot, but I do not move, not even to scratch my nose or hug myself against the wind. It seems natural that I should be there, although the storm is fierce and the lightning moves closer across the grass, great white arms of it lashing toward the ground from the high thunderheads. Then suddenly a quick series of bolts hits the ground, and the grass is branded in a circle not far in front of me. Again, on the far side of this burned patch, the long strands of electricity descend in a blinding circular curtain. As they lift, a man emerges from the smoke and walks away toward the far trees. I marvel. Where did he come from? How did he survive the lightning? Should I call out to see if he is okay? But I do not. I watch him recede, the now sky-bound crackles of light giving me glimpses as the stranger heads into the woods. That is all.

Gradually, I wake up.

Every now and then, like any chronic depressive, I find myself almost too tired to exist. For a long time, these periods frightened me, for I feared that I would do myself some harm in them. Even so, I did not identify with those others who attempted or threatened suicide, and I have come to see this as a failure on my part: at some level I thought that my burdens were greater, that my own longing for death was not the same as theirs.

In some ways, this is true. According to nature, after all, I *should* be dead. I have outlived the natural span of my life, and everything else has been extra. In other words, when I long to be dead, I am longing to be, in a sense, where I belong. Unlike a healthy person who commits suicide, so this line of thought goes, I would not be cheating fate or God or what have you. In fact, that is what I do by staying alive.

I am haunted by a story told me by one of my writing teachers. Driving many miles along a black and deserted road one night, Peter encountered an injured raccoon, apparently hit by a train or car, as it lay squirming in pain near some tracks that crossed the pavement in a low valley. Peter stopped the car and examined the animal, found its back broken and hind legs severed. He stood, anguished, looking around into the night as though help might arrive from somewhere. But it didn't and he knew it wouldn't, and so he decided to finish off the raccoon instead of leaving it to suffer. He got a two-by-four out of the back of the car and put all of his strength into a blow to the raccoon's skull. Years later, as he told me this story, his eyes glistened with tears. It had taken several strikes to kill the raccoon, even as badly injured as it already was, and Peter had been astounded at how difficult it was to do. "Life is determined," he noted, "and it holds on. It is really hard to kill something."

For me, however, it is not so. Rather than thinking of the active, violent difficulty of killing myself that images of suicide evoke, I think simply of ceasing all the effort required to keep me alive. It takes so much work to keep me here, especially to keep me feeling well enough even to want to be here. Every waking hour—and many of my sleeping ones—I am occupied with the labor of managing this disease. It pervades *everything*—getting up in the morning (am I coherent?), what kind of shoes I wear (and that determines greatly what kind of fashions I can adopt), who my friends are (because if someone cannot keep appointments, I can't tolerate her for long), what size carton of ice cream I buy (I don't want to have too much of it on hand), and—oh, just every little trivial decision. Testing blood sugar, taking insulin, preparing or obtaining appropriate meals at specific times, making sure that I exercise consistently (that means virtually every day), and the entire endeavor of continual self-monitoring take their chunk out of my schedule.

Some days it seems worth the effort, and some days it does not. When rewards are granted, when the air is good, the writing goes well, my blood sugar is stable enough that I am alert and calm, when a flock of yellow-rumped warblers flutters in the trees outside my windows, when the cat purrs and the bread rises fragrant and smooth, when a letter arrives, or a friend calls, or a new love flickers, then the work seems like no big deal. But let the yeast fail, the silence expand too far, the rain fall for days on end, the cedar waxwings in droves break their necks against the reflecting glass of an office building, the newspaper project too many headlines about children covered in cigarette burns, or the cat vomit on the rug, and I become overwhelmed, exhausted, and I resent the extra effort it takes to keep me going through what seems to be a pointless day. This used to drive me to distraction—and my friends and family as well. They, too, used to think I would try to hurt myself.

I don't think it will ever come to that, however. As I've grown less fearful of my longing for death, it threatens me less in actuality. In order to disarm the sensation, I really had to accept it, to cease fleeing from it, as from my fear of Kay, of blindness, of all those unknown things. I've come to see the longing for erasure as perfectly natural for someone who knows as much about the end as I do, who carries an extra load. Now, I simply take those feelings as a sign that I am tired, that I need to say no to some requests, that I need to remember that I can improve almost any day by being kind to myself.

When I first described these feelings to my brother, he expressed alarm, and, though I tried to reassure him that it had become more an interesting phenomenon than anything else, he wondered if I shouldn't turn myself in. A couple of weeks later, however, he called to say he'd had some insight, and it had come, strangely enough, from a television show about the Holocaust. "There was one still photo they showed," he told me, "of a concentration camp survivor as he stood on board a ship heading away from Germany. The look on his face was exactly the feeling you described."

"What did it look like?" I asked.

"As though he'd had a foot in some world beyond, and that it was hard to be sure he was back. It was in his eyes, a vision of the far away, a knowledge of death that couldn't be erased by any amount of good food and rest, and that would forever set him apart from those without the experience.

"I think," Kelly said, "that now I know what you mean."

That day the effort seemed worthwhile, as pleasant as breathing in the smell of a freshly baking loaf that your hands are still tired from kneading.

My struggle continues, never ending. I go back repeatedly to The Year—the loss of my rare friends because we moved across the state, the broken bones, the diabetes, the onset of menstruation, the rising tensions in my parents' marriage, the death of my beloved grandfather—and to my first depression, described to my old friends in numerous letters of the time. Mired in a complex web of unknown meaning and embarrassing weakness, my little girl's body now glows in memory with a pale vulnerability greater than that of the underbelly of a gazelle or of a crystal goblet tissued into a box for the rough ride on a moving van. How did I survive at all? And why is the world so stingy with its understanding? Would more sympathy merely have slid into pity and humiliated me? Wasn't its lack a sign of respect? Even now, as I write, there is a voice telling me to quit complaining, to be grateful for the sympathy and love I have had, which has been in no small measure.

So, I pose another, more inward question, Why is it never enough? Perhaps there is nothing that can make up for the injustice of a child being stricken by serious disease. However, there is something else which perhaps replaces that—a gleaming, clear light shed on the world. What it illuminates is not always pretty, but it is true, and in the warmth of that light I begin to cease mourning my long-gone innocence. Now, I understand my difference as a reason for living, dark chocolate as richer than milk and unsweetened mole sauce tangiest of all.

9

Avoiding Complications

On a glowing summer day shortly before my boyfriend Bill was to leave Pennsylvania for his new faculty position at the University of Washington, we sat around at a lazy barbecue basking in the warmth of the afternoon. A loose group of guys from Bill's department and the occasional female spouse or friend, we listened to the burgers sizzle on the grill, clanked our beers against the concrete patio, and sprawled on the shady lawn all around. Already I was apprehensive about Bill's departure, but that day seemed charmed—I felt welcomed into the by now familiar group, almost at home with the talk of baseball and lab processes and with the intermittent crudeness of the jokes. Much of it wasn't exactly my thing, but I felt I was learning to relax, to act normal, to hang out.

Then one guy began to describe his recent encounter with Cindy, one of the few women in the lab. She had been, he said, bleary-eyed and frantic, and she'd bitten his head off for getting in her way, then had tried to make excuses for herself by explaining that her cat was sick. "I guess she'd gone home the day before and found it completely catatonic," he said, elbowing a neighbor and chuckling at his pun.

"Was that Wednesday?" asked Joe. "I think she wasn't sure if it was going to live that day. I guess it had a stroke or something, but it's better now." He eyed me, knowing me as a cat lover.

The first guy nodded. "Yeah, yeah, I guess I should be more sympathetic. But, hell, it's just a cat. I mean, don't get me wrong—I like cats—but, hey, they're cats. When they die, they die. It's no big deal."

I felt Bill's hand run down my spine, as though to keep me calm, in line, well behaved, and I cringed slightly.

"You'd think it mighty strange if Bill and I broke up and I wasn't upset, wouldn't you?" I asked the cat-liker.

"Of course." He looked confusedly from my face to Bill's, unsure where I was going, not yet seeing any connection.

"You'd even expect me to cry?" I smiled coyly, beaming into his eyes, and turned my head to the side rather sadly. "Maybe even more than once?"

He nodded and shrugged, losing interest in what seemed like an irrelevant change of subject.

"Well, I've had my two cats for twelve years, that's eleven years longer than I've known Bill, so I don't think I'd be out of line to be upset if one of them was sick or dying. They've been with me through at least four men," I went on, "always right there through thick and thin. Why should the men be so much more important?"

The guy laughed. "Got me," he said. "But I still think people are different."

Indeed, they are. As I sat unsuspectingly at this barbecue, Bill's friends knew a lot that they weren't spilling. Later, after I'd uncovered his years and years of cheating on one girlfriend after another, his displaying this fact to his colleagues by doing so at every biochemistry conference the world over, and his own carrying on behind my back with at least four women, I would wonder what the hell they were thinking. Bill's lying at least had a clear cause, but the fact that all of them insisted on "minding their own business" meant that when I found out about Bill, I had to part with them as well, even Joe, who finally broke down and told me what was going on. I'd thought him a friend, but he'd watched Bill's cheating and lying for months without a word to me, and I'd had to confront him directly before he'd say anything. By that time, he hated Bill, but he clearly didn't care much about me either. He could have saved me a wasted year of my short life, but instead he minded his own business.

Though I've come to expect such deviations in myself from group values, even to appreciate my own strangeness, there is a righteousness implied here that is only occasionally a part of how I feel. The other side is that it is painful for me to be different, and to be so in such a remote way, without *looking* unlike the norms of my social groups. Most of the time, difference is obvious in some way—a person of color in a roomful of whites, someone in a wheelchair trying to negotiate a hallway swarming with legs and feet. That kind of difference has its own, perhaps even greater pains, but they are pains more readily acknowledged because they are visible and therefore verifiable from the outside. The normal folk seem responsible for exclusions in such situations, whereas with me, with this invisible difference of diabetes, I feel as though I create the problem myself. I am always trying to protect myself from the exclusions of others—because for me they come later, just when I'm beginning to feel accepted. Then I am unable to tell myself that my disability is the barrier, that if only these others would get to know me they would like me. That kind of defense may not eliminate the sting for the disabled or gay or other victim of unfounded prejudice, but I don't even have that thin bolster. It doesn't matter that it is often really my health that becomes the barrier between me and my loved ones because it doesn't *look* as though people reject me because of their own fear of my diabetes; it appears that they only reject me as one quirky individual. They need not even acknowledge their own prejudice or name it.

Once my friend Charlene complained that people in this largely white town were always assuming that everything was different for her because she was African American. "They seem to think that I'm from outer space," she said, "that just because I'm black they can't even invite me to dinner without asking if I eat *fish*."

"That's because you're a picky eater," I said, elbowing her, "not because you're black."

"Well, you know what I mean. When my niece came to live with me, all the neighbors kept saying how 'interesting' that was. 'It must be hard,' they'd say, 'but you people have different attitudes about that sort of thing.' That made me so mad—not all black people would take her in, not all white people wouldn't. And then there was the whole thing with the quote-unquote *holidays*. Do you know that Jerry had the nerve to ask me if 'you people' celebrate Christmas?" She shook her head. "I just get so tired of being the official representative of this exotic black culture. Every time there's a *diversity* issue, I have to go to the meetings. Sometimes I just want to say, 'You go. It's not that big a deal. We're not all that different, you know.' I mean"—she grinned—"we all pee the same way. And we *do* know what toilet paper is for."

We laughed. "It's funny," I said, "that you hate how they're always assuming you're different. I have just the opposite problem. Just because I look like any other white chick, they all assume I'm just like them, and then I have to listen to the most offensive junk about political candidates and cars and Tupperware parties."

That spring I designed a T-shirt for Charlene's extensive family reunion, and she gave me an extra shirt in return. It was one of our favorite things to wear them at the same time, to sit side by side on the exercise bikes, pedaling away, emblazoned as members of the same family, one chocolate brown and one pale pink, two sisters in alienation receiving like royalty the startled stares of those around us. With that T-shirt, Charlene helped me declare my own difference, but I also became aware of how necessary it was for me to do so myself—before my acquaintances assume that I'm just like them.

Otherwise, as has often happened, I end up where I don't belong. I invest in groups where ultimately I will be unable to remain, unable to accept the gap between them and me. Like most everyone, I long for affirmation, some sense of community or the love of an individual that buoys me when my confidence is low, or when my vision seems skewed and uncertain. Repeatedly I have latched on to some small commonality, only to find down the road immense chug holes, deep puddles, and ravines spanned by no bridge. The lock-stock-and-barrel nature of so many communities makes me flinch, and blanch, and eventually withdraw. I briefly dated a guy who appealed to me for his moral sense, his wish to be a positive force, but even if we had not parted when we did we eventually would have, for I never would have been able to bear the ersatz New Age spirituality of him and his alternative-healing community. The paradigm was so complete, every part in its place, everything happening for some unknown reason, and there seemed to me no room for the truly mysterious, the irrational, the ragged edge. That John could go to India to volunteer in an orphanage and then come home to his Ford Explorer and say that whatever happens is right and purposeful made me queasy. Of course, I never told him so, though I did argue my abstract belief in the accidental.

When one finds no niche, has spent one's life as a lonely individualist, it can be easy to invest way too much in relationships that are doomed. With Tad, as with Bill, I became a part of a social milieu that I found mostly infantile and perverse. I kept thinking that I'd get to know people better, or that I didn't have to like everyone or everything that went on in his group of friends. So, one friend was dealing drugs. So, one friend paraded her new lover in front of her old lover. So, she made a constant display of her belly and her sexuality, sleeping with one after another of the guys in the group. So, the guys made stupid comments about the allure of twenty-two-year-olds. So, one of them, finally looking for his first job at age thirty-three, refused to learn how to drive a car. I made endless excuses for my dislike of them simply because I loved certain things about Tad and because I wanted to find some community I could stand to be a part of. That was certainly not the one.

But by now I doubt the existence of one that will suit me. From my childhood days on the playground—when my two best friends were Susie, the Southern Baptist minister's daughter, whose family disparaged blacks and outlawed dancing, and Suzette, black as coal with a laugh like a bubbling stream—I have had individual rather than group friendships. Some of these have been very close and have lasted years, but those friends usually have groups to which they belong, to which their strongest bonds are forged. I remain, at least it seems to me, a sometime friend, an occasional lunch partner, a peripheral item. With few exceptions, those who are dearest to me always seem to have others who are more important to them. No wonder.

My friend and former housemate Craig is a case in point. I met him in 1987, when I first moved to Pennsylvania with Michael, and through all of the chaos of the years immediately following he remained a devoted friend. He still is. He shared a house companionably with me, he stuck by me when I was condemned by the gossip in the department he shared with Michael and Panos, and he now lets me sleep on his couch when I'm in New York. But I am not a member of the core group of friends-like-family that he formed when he was in grad school here: Shannon, Jennifer, and Mark make up the other terms in that equation. This is not their fault, and I do not blame them for leaving me out. I am glad that I have found a spot within their sphere at all, but I wonder where I was when their bonding was taking place. What was I doing instead?

Partly it happened because of the fact that Craig, Shannon, and Jennifer all shared a graduate school moment, but there are others who did so who, like me, remain on the periphery of the group, and there is Mark, who did not, at the center. Partly, it was because I threw myself into sordid and all-consuming love affairs that, by their suffocating domination over my ever-anxious mind, rendered me distracted from everything else. But it also can be attributed to my own assumptions: I got close and then no closer. I did not throw my lot in with theirs.

Craig and I lived together for one year while he worked on his dissertation and I labored to get over Panos and find an alternative future to working for the Penn State alumni magazine. In the spring, I declared that I would be leaving town by the end of the summer, and I began interviewing for jobs in Washington. The first trouble was that the jobs weren't, by and large, any more interesting than the one I had, and I began to formulate the idea that maybe I should try graduate school myself. The second trouble was that, by the time I made up my mind to stay, Craig had found another roommate, Shannon. I scrambled to find another apartment, but to no avail with my cats and my washing machine and my limited budget. In a couple of weeks, I would not only be working full-time but would be enrolled in a graduate workshop, my first, in which I desperately needed to impress my professor. Craig said that by no means would he and Shannon put me on a street corner, but I didn't feel secure enough, or capable enough to deal with the situation, to be comfortable with that. Out of fear and weariness, I told him that since the lease was in my name I wasn't going to move.

How on earth did I do such a thing? Here I had an offer—we're all in this together, we'll work it out somehow—and I withdrew into myself, protectively, individually, foolishly. Craig and Shannon ended up living close to campus in a large house with a third housemate, while I stayed in the neighboring town with a new roommate gotten through a newspaper ad, a guy so dumb we could hardly have a conversation. Miraculously, Craig forgave me, but I had absented myself from the scenes of friendship, from the household where over the years their tightest bonds were formed. When I think of what feelings led me to cut myself off this way, all I can think of are the exhausting requirements of my daily life, my need for control over my environment, and my fear of being cheated out of what should be rightfully mine. In retrospect, these seem ridiculous, poor excuses, but when I am in a tight spot they clobber me. It matters not that the blade is dull, it still severs.

. . .

And so, my friends love me, but from outside the barbed wire. Inside its sharp-tipped circle, I wave my greetings to them, but many of my friendships—though perhaps no more than usual in the course of a life—fail. What is unusual is that I grieve endlessly, each loss like missing pieces of a jigsaw puzzle, like holes in the distant landscape around my fence-enclosed prison. Seldom is anyone close enough to me to block out the spotty, Swiss-cheesy view all around, and when someone does come inside the wire he never stays long. No man has ever made a commitment of love to me.

Thank God, it is not as though I have remained a wallflower my entire life—I go over in my mind a litany of compliments from those who have admired me, the list of adventures and moments when I was sought after—but, again, there is some wall that I encounter. I look around some days in amazement at how everyone seems to be able to find someone right, but there isn't anyone right for me. A couple of years ago, I met a rather brash guy at a party, who voiced what others often think: "How is it that you've never been married?" he asked me insistently. "You look all right. What's wrong with you?"

There must be something wrong. Even though I am often plied with encouragement, with denials from friends and family, we still always try to figure out what is wrong with me. "You're fine, you're beautiful," my mother tells me, but she always tries to fix me up with older men who are uglier than proverbial sin. "You just haven't met the right guy yet," Rose once said, but two days later she was telling me that I should let my hair grow long in order to find the right kind of guy. "Quit wearing those baggy sweaters," Suzanne fusses. My boyfriends fall in love so hard that they nearly crack their faces on the sidewalk, but as soon as I open the door they're fleeing down the back alley, eyes on the horizon. "You're too intense," they call out as they go.

My own immediate family often flees from my presence and my problems. Every member of my nuclear family now has a new and separate family, but I have been unable to find a replacement, and I firmly believe that this is because I am "too much trouble." Since the year I was diagnosed, only one of my lovers and none of my friends and family has ever bothered to go out and buy a single book on diabetes. I handle it perhaps too well on my own, and even when I need help and assistance I am probably not grateful enough. I am dependent with an independent personality, and this attracts the wrong kind of people for bravery and loving care.

Recently in a conversation with my mother, I brought up the other-family phenomenon—my brother's marriage into an all-consuming New England clan; my father's flight to a second wife with a Laker Girl for a stepdaughter; and my mom's own second husband and, after his death, third husband and their kids and grandkids—and asked her what she thought about the idea that my diabetes was a major factor in the eventual breakup of my family and its re-creation in others. "Absurd," she said. "You know, when the parents of small children get divorced, the kids often think it's their fault. Maybe that same thing is going on here." I tried to hedge by saying that I don't think it was my fault, but that it had to do with how we never quite pulled together, we never talked about the emotional aspects of the disease. In a practical sense, we took care of it, but I view my family now, in that oh-so-clear hindsight, as completely overwhelmed and not particularly adept.

I don't mean to criticize my parents, for I am well aware of how much better than the run of parents they were and continue to be. My mother was sometimes obnoxious in her Pollyanna attitude, and my father's grouchy spells sometimes marred otherwise harmonious moments, but my parents were generally supportive, concerned, fair, and responsible. They educated us, far beyond what our schools provided; they clothed and fed and played with us; they tried to make each of us proud of our different talents. Somehow, though, we all intellectualized, and our affection usually was expressed in conversation, even debate. I didn't realize until years later that something—something physical—was missing for me: a whole range of bodily intimacy in terms of hugs and kisses and back rubs, in terms of instruction about the female vanities, but also in terms of learning how to swim and ride a bike, how to coordinate with others in team sports, how to dare to try new moves and bear the scraped knees and elbows of falling and trying again and falling once more. Even among us geeky academic types, I remain relatively timid and uncoordinated. I hike and jog and lift weights, but am afraid of rock climbing, cycling, sailing, downhill skiing, water skiing, ice skating, scuba diving, softball, Frisbee, volleyball, and a million and one other activities that most people share in tight little groups of rousing good fun. I tell my friends that I use up all my tolerance for pain, all my physical bravado, sticking needles and lancets in my belly and fingers, but really it's just that I don't inhabit my body the way most people do. I am too self-conscious.

Take up hobbies, goes the standard advice for the lonely. So I start concentrating on African violets and cacti, on caring for stray cats at an animal shelter—not the kinds of hobbies that allow for that kind of "being together" through which people seem to bond best and most easily. My family went camping together—we waded in streams and walked around nature trails and set up the tent and built campfires—but we did not go to the pool or ride bikes or spend weekends boating at the lake the way so many of my friends' families did.

Certainly, I can't list my parents' reasons for this, but can only speculate about their concentration on a pursuit of higher education—my father completing his doctorate when I was eight and my mother the year I graduated high school; their financial saving for my brother's and my own future educations; the interruptions to their own primary family togetherness—my father's parents divorcing when he was a child and his being sent to military school at age eleven, my maternal grandmother's nervous breakdown when my mom was twelve—and the consequent focus turned to parent instead of child. When I think back, though, I remember a shame about my body—whether silently communicated by my worried parents or simply something they were powerless to prevent being taught me by other sources, I don't know. It was a shame based upon a flaw and a need, an inferiority that I could never overcome.

But my diabetes happened to my family as well as to me, and perhaps even more than we ignored my feelings about it, we ignored theirs: my mother's determination that she had to make it all okay; my father's defensive stress about his career choices and the added financial burden, as though nothing he did would ever be enough; my brother's passivity in the face of sometimes unfair demands upon him. To this day I would venture that these emotional positions still characterize my family members. Maybe they would anyway, perhaps they already did when I was diagnosed, but the clear heightening of them all at that time is, I think, important. Not only did they not express how they felt about my having the disease, they also ignored feelings about having to deal with it themselves. None of them ever allowed themselves a little bit of resentment, which is too bad, as it might have been something we could have shared.

Perhaps, I think today, if we had more openly ranted and raged at my diabetes, it would not have weighed each of us down, would not have divided us ever so subtly the way anything unsaid produces a crack that may widen over the years. Of course, it is also possible that more expressiveness on my family's part would have hurt me, made me crazy. There is no way to know. However, I do see my disease's impact on those around me. Today my brilliant brother—of the National Merit and Presidential scholarships, the straight-A average, the Harvard degree, of all the potential in the world—is stuck in a lucrative but dull computer programming job; perhaps I sucked away the parental concern that might have encouraged him to try riskier ground. In his new family, with his wife and daughter and in-laws, he plays a caretaker role, and sometimes I see him putting their desires and values before his. Perhaps that only means he is a good husband and father, but nonetheless I speculate that he learned a certain acquiescence from living with the demands of my illness. My father, who has fortunately mellowed, still needs a lot of reassurance from me that I appreciate him, that I am grateful for his help. And my long-suffering mother, who recoils in guilt when I'm depressed, calls me every morning to make sure that I have not slipped into hypoglycemic shock during the night.

The thing is that I am supposed to be married by now, to have transferred my dependence from mommy to hubby. Why I haven't done so remains a great unknown: my family members, my friends, my shrinks, even my ex-boyfriends express surprise at this fact. It matters not how often they tell me how wonderful, even sometimes how beautiful I am. It matters not that I have had my fair share of lovers, or that there have been times when I've felt in demand, magnetic, sought after. What matters is that instantly upon my diagnosis, some stereotype of the ailing welled in my mind: asexual, out of style, humorless, conservative, abhorrent.

At that age I had no secure sense of myself as anything else—
that all depended on others—and I wasted my youth trying to
avoid being an out-of-it invalid. Still, many diabetics diagnosed
in their adolescent years do get married, even happily, and I have
not. I vacillate now between continuing to hope that I still may,
reminding myself that social norms don't have to control me,
trying to figure out alternatives for a sense of community, and
leaning backward on my mother.

My mother and I are both ashamed of her daily wake-up calls,
in spite of the fact that it is eminently practical and a minimal
part of each of our days. Other options—an aide dog, a computer
check-in service, possible death from insulin shock—seem even
less agreeable, either too time-consuming right now, too expensive, or too risky. Yet we despise the abnormality, and my mother
tires of the responsibility. Sometimes, when she forgets to call on
time, the sweaty guilt in her voice overwhelms me. Her husband,
though he has now informed himself about the seriousness of my
disease and is more sympathetic, is irritated by the demands this,
and my emotional ups and downs, place on her. She makes a
habit of calling me in private, out of his earshot. It is too much to
ask, that she be in charge, from so many miles away, of making
sure that I'm alive, but I ask her to do it.

Others, too, must participate in this ritual of abnormality.
Should I fail to answer the phone at 7:30 A.M., or should I answer
incoherently, my mother has a list of friends here in town who
have keys to my apartment and who have agreed to come and
save me. This being a transient town, and my relationships here
having been mostly ephemeral, some of these people don't know
me all that well, but I owe them my theoretical life. Though I'm
fond of the summer night breezes on my skin, I seldom sleep
naked when I'm alone, for it would be even more dreadful if I

were unable to cover myself up before Carolyn, or Don John, or Suzanne, or Leslee had to pump me full of emergency glucose.

It is even worse where lovers are concerned. Imagine the instant implications of my potential dependence, the relatively strict schedule of my meals, the occasional interruptions of romance due to low blood sugar, my restless sleep habits, and the plain fact that my body calls attention to its imperfections all the time. They have tended to feel that my dependence on them was something special, that it had to do with the particular relationship, that it meant that I wanted immediately all the commitments of marriage. Not. But they never believe this when I explain that my need extends to anyone who is near when it arises—parent, friend, stranger. And it is true that some people use illness to trap others: I think of a woman who recently posted to an electronic bulletin board I sometimes read. Her diabetic husband had such poor control over his diabetes and had become subject to such frequent undetected hypoglycemic episodes that she felt she could not leave him alone at home for more than a couple of hours. Even though I am not that way, the fear that I could be always haunts me and my lovers. Such nonexistent but phantom, implied, possible, threatened desperation renders me unable to say no to whatever demands my boyfriends have made. Someday he might save my life, so how can I say no to his little drinking problem, his subtly nasty remarks, his lack of punctuality, his very reasonable fear of me?

This situation seems to me sometimes as though it renders love and friendship untenable. It is an element that tips the scale away from intimacy by the sheer force of its enormous weight. Not even so much for others—they are usually glad to be of help, proud to be trusted—but for me. I don't want to owe them, I don't want the complications of the added burdens they might ask me to take on in return, I don't want to be a helpless invalid. Every complication—whether a physical effect of the diabetes, such as cataracts and gastroparesis, or the demand that any other needy person might make and that I might fail to meet—threatens me with failure.

After I moved from Tennessee to Minnesota for college, I used to say that I liked living in the North better than in the South, not so much because I liked the North better, but because I could name an excuse for my frequent alienation. In the North, when I felt estranged from those around me, I could tell myself it was because they were all a bunch of yankees, but when I experienced this sense of oddness at home, I had no excuse for it. It just meant that I was weird. Today, I've come to naming my diabetes, a natural progression from having to explain how many things I do are determined by it.

In the gym, when some helpful guy begins advising me about how to increase the weights I lift, I tell him that it's a diabetic thing—I have to use smaller weights to reduce the risk of blood vessels exploding in my retinas.

When I can't run my usual miles with a friend, I have to explain that it's a diabetic thing—the variations in my blood sugar can wreck my workouts, dramatically alter my performance from day to day.

When I indulge in the luxury of having my legs waxed, I respond to the inevitable surprise that such a blond thing as me should have such dark and prolific thigh hair (defensively, because I don't want to be accused of being a fake blonde) that it's a diabetic thing—we will grow dark hair wherever there is a follicle that will do so.

The little tire around my middle? It's a diabetic thing—frequent injections to one area often cause this hyperlipotrophy, or extra deposits of fat cells. It will never go away, no matter how many sit-ups I do, though I could try harder.

As I sit shivering in my group therapy sessions, and my psychologist reaches to turn up the heat, I say, "No. I'll be cold sitting here no matter how warm the room is. It's a diabetic circulatory thing."

My extra sinus infections, my numerous yeast infections, last spring's kidney infection—all of them, I remind people, are diabetic things. I have to eat right, I have to take my medications, I have to go to the doctor more often than they do.

For a graduate student, I spend a lot of money on certain things, and these, too, I justify by my diabetes: seeing an ophthalmologist rather than an optometrist, having my teeth cleaned every three months, buying expensive shoes, joining a gym where I can work out on my schedule, paying for fresh fruit and vegetables year-round. Others may see these as indulgences, but they are diabetic things.

The times that I freak out and get angry when someone is late are a diabetic thing—I need to eat on time, I need to know where the next meal is coming from, I need to be able to count on something. When I suddenly grow weary at a party, when I'm shaky and irritable with excess norepinephrine pounding through my body after a low, when I "go stupid" and inattentive—yes, yes, these, too, often come from diabetes.

All these complications of diabetes I have tried to avoid, to no avail. It is a diabetic thing, I explain, for the ravages to be implacable.

This may be but a phase, and I may return again to not using it as an excuse. Right now, however, it feels just fine to do so, to allow myself the protection from expectation that being defined by it affords me. This is just the opposite, I realize, of what is supposed to be emotionally sound, but even though I find no like-minded cadre of individuals in the community of diabetes—we are not passionate about the same things; we are not drawn together by politicization of our condition—I like noting the parallels between diabetes and the other parameters of my belief and behavior. Like my glucose readings, which I must keep in a narrow middle range, I find myself oddly bound by beliefs that keep me between camps. I've no religious proscriptions against premarital sex, but I think promiscuity and cheating are revolting and degrading to everyone involved. I'm pro-choice, but think that feminist advocates have missed the boat by not addressing the real moral issue of the fetus's life. Wedding ceremonies often make me cringe with their incipient sexism, but I long to be publicly and spiritually married. I have a radical sensibility, but I like to eat dinner at seven every night. I belong neither in the world of selfish and empty alternative lifestyles pursued by so many nontraditionalists of my generation nor in the often smug universe of the absolutely traditional. Perhaps I just chalk all of this up to my diabetes because it's convenient, but ironically it allows me more ease with others whom I used to condemn or feel alienated from.

I can now see that the fear that I invoke in myself and others is not about all of me. I could not be flexible with my friend Rose about running schedules because of my diabetes. Tad grew determined to develop our relationship no further right after an episode in which he had to revive me from hypoglycemia. My mother gets weary of my diabetes, not of me. Others carry such a burden for my life, but the burden that weighs on me is reminding them constantly of how inseparable my diabetes is from me. If this turns them away, so be it.

A great cosmic no was shouted to me at age eleven, and there always hovers over me a hand that waits to pluck security and happiness away each time they come to me. I have grown up in the looming shadow of that hand, and I seem unable to escape it. To others this hand may seem imaginary, and some of them name my attitude as the source of my grief and losses—if only I would move out from under the shadow of the hand, or better yet simply erase it, all would be fine. To them, I say that sometimes our fates are not of our choosing. The world has not been gentle with me. Though I have stumbled across a good many wonderful things, I have not found the niche I have sought, and I have searched hard. I cannot get rid of the shadow of the hand. That there is no one to blame, no reason, makes this all the more enigmatic, like blind people who can see into others' minds, like children who passingly make the wisest observations, like a cat who puts her soft paw on your cheek when the tears slip from your lashes and no other human is there to comfort you.

10

Cassie's Shots

In the spring of 1996 my Cassie Marie came down with diabetes. One of the two venerable cats—going on fifteen years old—that I'd gotten shortly after graduating from college, Cassie was as close to me as meringue on a pie. At a year old, she'd collided with a car, and I had nursed her through several weeks of broken hip, shattered pelvis, and incontinence. We had the kind of bond produced when an animal learns to wait until you hold her over the kitty litter before she will pee. Though she often disapproved, as cats will, she trusted me almost completely. So when diabetes befell her, she offered no resistance to my ministrations. Instead, with a look of patient annoyance in her half-flattened ears and her narrowed green eyes, she would jump up to the place I patted on the end of the bed and wait for her injection. She was lucky, I suppose, in that I knew what I was doing. The veterinarian had been frankly delighted that, when she had begun to explain that diabetes was treatable in cats, that it only required an injection a day—of a kind of insulin called "regular" and which I could get at any pharmacy with her prescription—I replied I already had both regular insulin and syringes at home. In spite of some mild embarrassment, she could not hide her grin. "That makes it a lot easier for me," she said. "A lot of people refuse to do it, especially at first. Just a few weeks ago, a couple said they'd just take the cat home and let it die 'peacefully.' Fortunately, they changed their minds as they watched her deteriorate, but it was a shame that she had to suffer those weeks." She smiled ruefully, and I remembered my childhood sensation of being too much trouble, of wondering if I might not, too, be allowed to die, even euthanized.

There was no question, of course, that I would treat Cassie's diabetes, tedious and painful though it might be. Keeping her around definitely seemed worth the trouble, though I hated giving her shots seemingly more than she hated receiving them, and my hands shook just as they had when I'd first learned to dose myself. Then, too, that the cat of a diabetic person should become diabetic seemed bizarre, somehow karmic and fateful, as though the disease were so woven into my existence that even creatures near me could not escape it. I felt guilty, as though contagious somehow, as though God felt it necessary to demonstrate to me an iota of how my parents had felt when saddled with my illness. Never, never, I thought, will I be able to escape this sensation of punishment—either divine retribution for some unknown sin or an unfair penalty for no crimes committed at all, from an arbitrary god that followed no logic but merely lashed out incoherently. I had no idea where this sense of punishment had come from—I was not Catholic, after all, or even a fundamentalist Protestant—and I even considered it borderline kooky, but I continued to feel that it was somehow just not all right for me to be who I was. Everything bad was my fault. Feeling terribly responsible, I wanted only to stay at home with Cassie, to make sure that she was okay. However, over the next few months, she, in her simple little animal way, would demonstrate that, in fact, we were in it together, that I was certainly not alone with the responsibility. She had already had a rough eight months of health problems, and the next year would be even harder.

The previous August Cassie and her sister Stella had picked up a few fleas from my mother's dog, the problem being that they were allergic to fleas and the literal few could wreak havoc, with the cats chewing themselves into a frenzy of sores and hairless spots in a matter of days. This time, the original two fleas must certainly have been on Cassie, for Stella seemed fine, and for this reason the vet interpreted Cassie's rash as an allergy to something else—ragweed or some such. He gave her a shot of steroids to alleviate the itching for a month and told me that by then the allergen would be gone. But after the temporary respite, Cassie began to bite and claw herself again, and by mid-October she was a mess. In spite of my asking about the possibility of fleas, the vet insisted that he could find none on her and gave her another steroid shot. He wanted to know if I had a new rug—no—and asserted that even if the windows were closed I could bring in enough fall pollen on my clothes to irritate the cat. But, but . . . the cat was fourteen and had never been so allergic to anything but fleas. Still, I bowed to his authority.

The middle of November arrived with one of the biggest and heaviest snowstorms I'd ever seen in central Pennsylvania, and when I awoke on the morning of the sixteenth, I found the box elder in the backyard lying across the top of my car like a weary giant sleeping in a tiny chair. There had been no crashing fall;

the tree had gradually sunk and split under two days' worth of steady, wet snow which had increased that night to a muffling blanket thick as a down comforter and heavier than armor. Cleanup would take the borough days and days—plowing and trucking away the volumes of snow, spreading salt on the ice, restoring power lines, clearing away the fallen trees that poked up everywhere through the crust like broken matchsticks—and I would not have transportation for nearly eight weeks while the roof of my car was being replaced.

By now it had become clear from the telltale trail of gritty brown dirt griming up their favorite napping spots that the cats did indeed have fleas. Both of them were scratching madly and puking up hairballs every other day, and I cursed both the vet and myself for being so stupid and letting this go on so long. I combed them with a flea comb and made another vet appointment for the Friday after Thanksgiving, when my mother would be visiting and could ferry us across town. Lo and behold, however, a receptionist called on Wednesday to let me know that they would not be open on Friday after all, mumbling some excuse about electrical repairs. My explanation that I would have a difficult time coordinating transport to their office the following week merited this reply: "Well, we're not open next week anyway because it's the opening of deer season, and Dr. Moss will be hunting."

"My cat is very sick," I said, my voice already quavering with outrage, "and Dr. Moss has not been very effective at treating her. I think he has some responsibility here. Isn't someone else going to handle his patients?"

"Only on an emergency basis," she said, clearly annoyed.

"Get my records ready for pickup," I told her. "I'll be changing vets." Dr. Moss had never been my favorite, though he had always been kind to the animals. For several years I had seen mainly his partner, Dr. Kleiman, whom I liked a good bit, but she had disappeared the previous year without any comment from him, and things at his office had been going downhill ever since. Sometimes no one answered the phone during regular hours; the usual receptionist had had a difficult pregnancy and had been replaced by middle-school kids and this officious temp; and now this.

My new vet was aghast and prescribed immediate pyrethrin baths and treatment of the house, as well as fatty acid capsules and antihistamines instead of steroids, which, she noted, could induce diabetes in a cat this age. By January, both cats were feeling much better, and I breathed freely and caught up on my other bills again, but by April Cassie exhibited the classic symptoms of diabetes: weight loss and frequent urination. She lapped up bowls of water and grew lethargic, barely even bothering to notice the buzzing flies of spring on the porch. Of course, I knew exactly what was wrong. I knew how distant the world must seem to her.

After Cassie and I had settled into our new morning routine— first my blood sugar test and injection, then her shot (no test, as it still takes venous blood for that in a cat)—a few weeks passed uneventfully. She acted her cheerful, obnoxious, demanding self again. Then one day, as I was dressing and getting ready to head to campus, she flopped off the end of the bed, hit the floor, and wobbled around the room. I treated her low blood sugar with instant glucose, she recovered, and I left for school, but when I returned home she was hiding under the bed, immobile, and when I picked her up, she peed a warm stream down my front and hung like a pocketbook in my hands. From this severe low she also recovered, and as it turned out her diabetes had been rescinded never to return.

Cassie, however, was beginning the process of dying.

. . .

Always, I have loved animals—dogs, cats, horses, and the whole panoply of more exotic pets and wild critters that I've never had the desire to touch, just to watch. Their familiar strangeness fascinates me, the way that I can communicate with them and yet they remain unknown and mysterious, hilarious and poignant, devoted and simultaneously alien and remote. Like me and not like me. In my memory, I wander dimly back down the dark hallway of the house we lived in, looking for the kid I was, a child who couldn't stand for any creature to suffer. From the living room, where I lay on the carpet eating Hershey's Kisses the day of my diagnosis, I could look out on the deck to where on a chilly February day our dog might curl up with the cat against the sliding glass door, and I might open that door and sneak both of them down that narrow hallway to my bedroom and close the door. The room is pink, with a hideous shag carpeting that doesn't match the heavy floral drapes, the old-fashioned four-poster bed, or the pretty Queen Anne–style secretary that had been a birthday gift from my parents. Everywhere there are animals—a pink stuffed teddy bear, china dogs from Walgreen's, a carved marble cat, a pottery mouse, a fur mouse with a leather tail, a whole collection of equine examples including a strange chocolate brown horse and foal in a soft velvety material with luxurious fake-hair manes and tails, a large plastic dun with a saddle I'd made myself, a tiny painted wooden specimen both delicate and square, racehorses cut from the newspaper, my favorite poster of an overgrown palomino Shetland captioned, "A forelock is like bangs." Our animals, my father decreed, must stay outside, but I had already busied myself with this secret life of bringing them in, the real live animals as well as the toy and paper ones. Our crazy gray cat named Lint gave birth to two different litters underneath my bed, and my sweet brown dog, Not Spot, often slept next to me on the bed. Her warm, pink-spotted tongue licked away many tears of fear I remember crying. Comforted by her wriggling warmth against me, I slept better. She didn't care what I looked like or that sometimes I cried. She didn't mind that I was ill and moody.

Who did? The truth is that I don't really remember any clear development of an aversion to hypochondria, a sense that others often believe that I overestimate the seriousness of the ups and downs of my disease. Small details flood my mind, all of them trifling, but all of them adding and adding and adding to each other:

My grandmother, her delicate fingers at her breast, disappearing into her bedroom whenever a responsibility arose that she found odious. She could, the doctor tattled, evoke her own arrhythmia, and every time thereafter that it happened, whispered resentments fluttered between family members like bloodsucking bats.

The hideously insulting depiction of the poor schmuck with allergies in *Sleepless in Seattle*. I hate that movie more than any other, simply because it implies that no one with a physical ailment could possibly be sexy or good enough for Meg Ryan. True love no longer includes that part about "in sickness and in health."

The mantra of the yoga class, the meditation circle, the alternative health publications, repeated over and over, that I am responsible for my own health, that I can heal myself, that I just need a positive outlook.

My own fear of telling my current physician any new set of minor symptoms that plague me. I have been seeing this doctor for ten years now, I know him as a good guy, he has never demeaned me, and we have hammered out a decent rapport, but

I still have to work myself up to justify "bothering" him with minor symptoms. Many times he does dismiss them, but why don't I feel that that's what he's there for? After all, how am I to know what is the first step on the downhill slide, what symptoms are meaningful and serious, and what I should be trying to catch early rather than late? Does this tightness in my chest indicate a stressful period or am I developing heart disease? Is it okay for my face to flush such deep red when I run? This diarrhea—is it gastroparesis? Every little twinge could drive me crazy if I let it, but why should I be so ashamed to check them out with my doctor?

I think of my college friend Audrey's high compliment that I didn't let the diabetes stop me from doing what I wanted, of Charlene's assertion when I was thirty that I did and shouldn't, of the ways in which I have isolated myself further these days, retreating into a private world where I can veil my need to sleep off the exhausting effects of frequent low blood sugars, where all my peculiar habits can have free range without anyone else making a comment about it. My health is worse than it used to be, but still I make it hard to see the ill effects.

Just today, in a meeting with a professor I'd never met before, I explained my interest in the ailments of certain famous writers with reference to my own long-term diabetes. "But you *look* so healthy," he said. "One would never suspect." That double-bind curse and compliment. I look healthy—great—but that also implies that it couldn't possibly be serious or painful or debilitating, that my reality is not quite real.

Animals are the only ones I trust never to evaluate me.

Mostly, however, I realize that the goad and judge are me. A couple of years ago, before my mother and I developed our daily call routine, there came one of those mornings when my blood sugar went so low that I almost didn't get up. When I finally came to, I was standing in the kitchen, staring at the dancing letters on a bag of cinnamon-apple Toasty O's, leaning over and cramming cereal into my mouth on automatic pilot. I jerked my head up and goggled around—cabinets gaped open, the refrigerator door breathed a crack of cold air into the already chill room, sugar from the overturned bowl sparkled across the floor. I recognized the letters on the cereal bag as something familiar, but I could not make sense of them, though I stared for a long time, as my jaws and throat did their thing unrelated to my brain. Then I blacked out again.

The next time I came to, I stood against the washing machine in the basement, shoving clothes into an already agitating, water-filled compartment. The sound of the machine shifting into wash mode, I think, had snapped me awake, and I knew, at least, that it was odd I was doing laundry. What day is it? I wondered. What am I doing here?

Desperately, I climbed the stairs back to the kitchen and surveyed the mess—milk still out, bowl and sugar bowl, spoon flung into the sink, bags and boxes strewn around. I wondered how much I had eaten, but also knew that I was lucky I'd done so at all. Barely, I could grasp where I had been, but that day coherence was for some reason particularly slow to return. I went upstairs to the bedroom and found the carton of orange juice on the bookcase, but still I just could not figure out the day. By then, I shivered with the delayed reaction I often have—turning freezing cold—and I crawled back under the covers to sleep. From outside the closed blinds, an eerie glare surrounded the house. I felt as though I slept in a science-fiction film, and soon enough I awoke again.

This time, I knew that responsibilities awaited me. What if I was supposed to be teaching a class? Worse yet, what if I were due to make a presentation in one of the courses I was taking? The general outline of my life grew clear, but I still had no idea what day it was. I pulled on my bathrobe and wandered the house trying to remember. Finally, I had the bright idea of looking at the list of to-do items I kept in the front of my calendar. Most of the tasks for Wednesday had been checked off, so that meant it had to be Thursday, and I was due in class at 9:00. I looked at the clock: 8:37. Shit.

I flew into a panic. This professor was a strict taskmaster, and it never occurred to me that it would be okay if I were late. No time for a shower, but I ran upstairs and ran cold water over my arms, splashed it across my cheeks, and brushed my teeth. When I tested my blood sugar, it had rebounded but only to 70 or so, despite the fact that I'd obviously eaten enough calories for a week. Should I take an injection now, when I still *felt* so low, or should I risk letting it bounce too high a little later? I threw my meter, syringes, and insulin in my bag and decided to take care of it on class break. The thought of going low again made my head pound. I gathered up my books and papers, shoved them in my bag, glanced one last time at my lopsided hair, and opened the front door.

To my dismay I discovered that the source of the glare, which I had somehow continued to manage to misunderstand, was a new foot of snow, freshly fallen and untouched by shovel or blower. I retreated again and pulled on my boots before blundering off through the drifting white powder, the time already 9:05 and me nearly a mile from campus. By then I was raging in my mind, the traces of the norepinephrine that had probably saved my life by getting me out of bed now filtering out into a jarring irritability and anger. I cursed my hard-nosed teacher—everything about her and her class. I hated my classmates, that brown-nosing, smooth-living, professionally demeanored crew that would sneer

at me when I arrived in such a tizzy. Of course, many of them
missed classes and canceled office hours whenever they had a little sniffle, but I had never allowed myself such an indulgence,
had, in fact, during five years of graduate school never missed
anything due to illness, though I had often felt like hell. The
Puritan writers we were studying in the course also came in for
my wrath, and I blamed them for every banal convention, such
as punctuality. No one, I was sure, would understand. If I told
them that I'd had a low blood sugar, they would simply go on as
though I'd said I'd sneezed—why, with less sympathy than if I'd
said I had a cold. By the time I arrived at the department at
around 9:25, I was sweating across brow and nose in spite of the
fierce wind and still-spitting snow and had worked myself into a
frenzy. Half an hour late—unbelievable!

A note on the seminar room door said: "English 542 will begin
at 10:00 today, due to the snow." Fury, dejection, embarrassment,
and relief collapsed me into a heap in a nearby chair, where I
then turned on myself. What a fool not to call. Of course
all those who lived driving distance away from campus, including my professor, would have to wait for the plows to make the
rounds. Why had this never occurred to me? Here I had strained
myself beyond belief—for nothing. I tried to calm myself,
to relax the marauding temper rather than just changing its target. At least no one would know. I wouldn't have to explain my
tardiness.

My bad morning, however, had not ended. As I trudged
upstairs to my office where I might pant in peace for the next half
hour, I paused at a bulletin board and was attacked by a woman, a
fellow student with whom I'd had some acrimonious professional
differences. Standing mute and groggy, I listened to her insult my
efforts as a representative on our graduate student board. "Maybe
next year," she said, "the group will do something worthwhile."

Usually, I didn't mind a good fight with her, but that day I merely nodded and slithered off like melting ice, the heat of her voice pulsating after me down the hall. Finally at my desk, in my tiny metal cubicle, I put my head down and let some tears trickle down my cheek. My God, I thought, I nearly died this morning and then I encountered her and that was worse. Even she would not have attacked me that way had she known what I'd just been through. The juxtaposition struck me, and I longed for a situation that would protect me when I'd been near death this way. No one could even tell, and even if I told, no one could quite believe it. Maybe I couldn't, either.

After Cassie recovered from her weeks with diabetes, she had a good summer. I packed up and took both the cats with me to Connecticut, where I was teaching in a summer writing program for high school students at Choate Rosemary Hall. Strangely enough, both the cats, but especially Cassie, seemed to enjoy the change of scene and settled right into the apartment I shared with my friend Sally, sashaying around as if they owned the place and cackling at the birds coming to the feeder outside the dining room window. By summer's end, however, I noted that Cassie was hardly eating a thing. She had shrunk to a teaspoon weight under all her fluffy fur.

Cassie had developed liver trouble, the vet explained, and that might actually have been what had given her the diabetes symptoms earlier. Short of a biopsy, which she was probably too old and weak to withstand anyway, there was no certain way of telling what was wrong with her liver—cancer, cirrhosis, one of several types of infection—but only one of these causes was really treatable anyhow, and so we treated her for that, a particular kind of long, slow infection that often recurs even when eradicated once. The treatment—five pills a day—would last a month, and during that time we wouldn't know if it was even appropriate, much less whether it was working.

That month stands out in my mind as one of the worst ever. I shoved huge pills down Cassie's throat until I thought the gagging would scar her, the way bulimics develop calluses on the roofs of their mouths from the repeated gouging of their fingernails. The antibiotics, of course, nauseated her, and she refused to eat unless I begged her to do it. Half the time she puked up the food shortly after eating. With minimal hope, I scooped up morsels of her favorite flavors, bits of leftover chicken and deli turkey, on the end of my forefinger and stuck it under her nose to smell. "Just a bite," I'd say. "Just one more little bite." She weighed barely four pounds, down from eleven in her prime. About halfway through the month, lying on the couch one night, we had a tête-à-tête in which she indicated that she herself was ready to go any time. She looked into my face, and her expression told me this: she was eating, living, carrying on, just to please me. I promised her that I would not put her through this again if the infection recurred, that I just wanted her to hang on through the rest of the month and see what happened.

Only so much suffering, I reflected, is worthwhile, even if there is the possibility of recovery. This little cat submitted to my ministrations quite docilely, but she had also, I could see, reached a point where it really didn't matter to her. It was an interesting and emotional thing to sense so clearly in her. There was nothing tentative or uncertain about it. Her life had been worth fighting for, worth, in my terms, a lot of trouble, but every life reaches a point where the sacrifice is not worth it, where the saved are only preserved in their own suffering, for the illusion upheld for others. I marveled that a *cat* could communicate this so unequivocally to me, when I am usually a person who begs more and more definition and refinement of articulation even when others speak

English. "What do you mean by that?" I ask all the time. Or I quibble about others' interpretations of my own words: "I didn't say *exactly* that," I say. "What I meant was more like this. . . ." I knew, however, precisely what my silent kitty wanted, though there was no explaining how.

In those weeks of nursing her, I received another clear insight, another gift from my animal companion: she made it completely obvious that my own suffering had never come close to the kind that makes life not worth living. I realized that I would know when that time came, if it came, and that I needn't worry about it anymore.

Amazingly enough, at the end of the month, Cassie's blood work looked good. Though there were still some signs of damage, her liver had recovered most of its function. Her appetite never fully recovered, but she eased on through the winter and gained another spring for rolling on the warm boards of the porch in the sunshine.

That first summer that I'd taught at Choate had been telling in a number of ways, not the least of which had to do with the fact that it was the first time I'd lived with anyone since my summer with Bill in Seattle—four full years. A fellow student in the M.F.A. program and a writer I admired more than the sky, Sally had been a friend for several years. Instantly upon moving into our sublet apartment at Choate, I became terrified that Sally would grow to hate me. At Choate, she was in her element— she had attended high school there, had taught there full-time right after college, and had designed the program in which we were teaching that summer. I knew nothing about high school students or the snooty private academy environment, and besides, I just wasn't as cool as Sally. I didn't wear the latest fashions on a stylishly thin body. I didn't have a ragged Harley-Davidson T-shirt or wildly curly hair in a halo around my face. I couldn't run marathons. Nor could I recite the entire history of rock 'n' roll and reggae or the full schedule of the upcoming college football and basketball seasons. I was afraid that living and working in such close proximity with me, Sally would find me boring and tedious, that I would run out of witty, entertaining things to say, that she would see through what I suddenly realized was a carefully constructed public persona, one which even my closest friends never got past. The entire first week and a half I spent trembling—the students would hate me, I wouldn't be able to teach them anything, the other teachers would hate me, they would never want to party with me, I'd be too tired anyway, Sally would be embarrassed by me, she would end up giving me a critical speech about what was wrong with me, how I needed to be, how my problems interfered with my happiness. She would do this, of course, out of a desire to help. All of this played through my mind like a movie, and though I was shocked at my own insecurity I could not stop it.

Sally, fortunately, is not a person who lets her observations stew long in her brain, and she is capable of taking responsibility for her own annoyance, so none of my worst fears came true. The apartment we shared contained as much space as a royal palace—two floors of an old house, complete with kitchen, dining room, living room, study, three bedrooms, and two baths—and so we each could retreat to a safety zone of privacy. Even more important, I trusted Sally enough to tell her how afraid I was. For her part, Sally made plenty of comments about me and who I am, but the fondness with which she did so validated our differences rather than expanding them.

One day, as we walked back to the house from our classrooms, trekking from the upper campus down a long hill past the I. M. Pei arts center, across Christian Street, then up a slight rise to the building housing the mail room, we rattled on about our students and what the plan for the next day would be. At the juncture of one driveway and Christian Street, a huge brown van squatted on the verge of a sharp dip in the pavement, engine running, its putative driver standing at the open back doors rummaging in a pile of gear and boxes. Blithely, Sally continued up the sidewalk.

"Let's go *behind* the van," I said, pulling her by the arm.

She stopped in her tracks, looked around, and said, "What are you talking about?"

"Who knows if that guy has put the parking brake on," I said. "Who knows if he's left the thing in gear. I don't want to get plastered to the pavement by some stupid van."

A grin lit up Sally's face. "You think of everything," she said. "Consequences. You always see all the potential consequences. You can see the future."

I blushed, as I had been really seen, but soon we laughed, and though Sally teased me repeatedly about my sensitivity to potential disaster, it was not a characteristic she found useless or stupid, even though it was as far from her own thinking as could be. Instead, she harnessed me to talk over all kinds of hypothetical situations related to Choate, to the books we wanted to write, to her marriage and her insistence on the importance of her friends, sometimes to her husband's dismay. We could talk about my prescience about consequences in relation both to my disease and to writing, for I find traditional plots incredibly predictable even when others are surprised by them. When the film *The Crying Game* came out, everyone seemed taken aback at the female who turned out to be male. Not me, I knew it early on. Ditto in terms of a fiction reading I went to recently—a well-known, well-published short story writer read a beautiful piece—the language and images were startling, but the two major plot surprises I found embarrassingly predictable. Sally and I could explore in conversation how my own interest in regular plots is minimal, how both my written stories and my life story have a different kind of plot, numerous subtle almost invisible connections, leaps, and seemingly irrelevant details. Amoebas—that's what I call my stories—and the tangled way that my diabetes oozes into all aspects of my life, I believe, contributes to that style, as it contributes to my style of thinking about consequences, about what is coming next, about where this road is going.

What made Sally capable of appreciating these qualities when others are usually so disturbed by them that they flee at the first real sight of me, I do not know, but the summer ended up being as much a pleasure for me as for the cats. I still worried from time to time; I still felt self-conscious about my periods of exhaustion in the face of Sally's incredible, driving energy; I still often wanted to hide my weaknesses behind closed doors. But for the first time in a long time, I also felt incredibly loved because Sally could actually see me—the real me—and still find value there. She didn't want to fix me, to make it all better, to correct my strange behavior. To her, I just was the way I was, a friend, a delight in all my difference. It had been a long time since I'd felt such affectionate recognition.

Cassie Marie lived another six months before her kidneys failed and I had her euthanized. When I returned home from a weekend trip in May of 1997, the sad and addled look had returned to her face, and my cat-sitter reported that although she had enjoyed sitting on the porch in the sun she wouldn't eat and seemed very weak. I whisked her off to the vet's, expecting the worst, which I got. Nothing could be done. She was too old for a kidney transplant, and even if she hadn't been I really couldn't afford to fly her to California for such experimental surgery. I took her home for what I hoped would be a last week of cuddles, but when she fell down the steps the next day I knew the end need be sooner. I made the appointment.

During the next twenty-four hours, her last, I tried to tempt her with all manner of treats and catnip, with turkey and tuna fish, but mostly what she wanted was to sit on my lap, to curl tiny but still warm against me, purring her remaining cosmic affirmation, so unafraid of death. On a Wednesday afternoon, I held her while the vet slipped the needle into her leg and the last remaining light disappeared from her eyes. I grieved, but knew that she had had the perfect life, and this, as well as my own ability to see her through to the end, filled me with a serene acceptance. Even her ashes, returned to me in a baggie tucked inside an ugly plaid tin, sparkled in the light—beautiful, dusty, gritty, eternal matter. I had *seen* Cassie—her flippant swishing of her fabulous tail, her grumpy disgust at the existence of dogs, the way she would pull out a drawer and climb up on the bathroom vanity waiting for me to turn on a drip of tap water, her favorite way to drink. She had been *known*, that silly creature, and therefore she had lived quite fully.

My own secretiveness, avoidance of rejection by hiding away the reality of my life, I know, keeps me from being really known, really loved. The struggle for me continues to be setting aside the perfectly reasonable and experience-confirmed fears and risking myself again and again. The alternative of self-protection makes of life a paltry thing, a television existence, a two-dimensional fright show, but it is tempting, tempting and peaceful. Writing about this is an attempt to change it, an interim way through this lonely time, a way to make myself visible without taking the bullets directly. Here on the page I can be both myself and my disease, without ignoring the latter or being subsumed by it, without subjecting myself to the fear I evoke in others. But I also want this off the page: to live as fully, to be as completely known, as my broken-boned, grouchy, roly-poly, little green-eyed cat. I abide with that hope, though it often seems to be to an empty room that I say, See? Here I am with all my flaws. See?

Others are afraid; I am afraid. I know that some of my current solitude is due to rejection, and some to self-protection. I also know that this phase, too, shall pass into a time when I will move more widely in the world again, going perhaps more easily back and forth between its standards and those of my own body. Still, even with the reality of my body so often invisible, somehow I will always stand, like the crude black-lettered, white-painted signs scattered along the highways of my Tennessee childhood, proclaiming that passersby should GET RIGHT WITH GOD or that THE END IS NEAR. Many people accelerate, whooshing in a rush by my kudzu-threatened face, my battered existence. Dear fools, I think to those who flee, leaving me alone in this rich and rigorous silence, you, too, are dying. Would it not be better to mark the interval together, looking at what is really here, seeing others, telling the truth about our bodies, neither so perfect as we might hope nor so horrible as we dread?

As the blithe healthy stream by, I wave, rooted here, solid and knowing, waiting for them all to come back this way someday soon. It is a fine, inevitable place. See?